DISCLAIMER

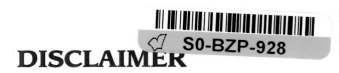

Media Perspectives
777 First Street, PML 163
Gilroy, CA 95020-4918

Introduction...

This book is the result of a survey that was sent out to plastic surgeons all throughout the US. This is not the opinion of the author, but the opinion of the doctors who participated in the survey. There are absolutely **no paid-for listings.** The vision for this book is to be a tool for you to use in the research process of finding a well trained and qualified plastic surgeon that will meet your needs. Although most the doctors who participated were certified by American Board of Plastic Surgeons (ABPS) (Please see Check Credentials for more information about ABPS) there may be doctors who were voted for and won best that are not certified by ABPS and or may not be classified as a plastic surgeon, but due to their skills in a certain procedure were noticed for their excellence.

When reviewing this book please keep in mind that only a few doctors could be listed as best but by no means does this mean that there are not equally gifted surgeons listed under the Doctors Specialty list. The cause of this may be several reasons. First, some doctors who's practice are not grouped around major hospitals may not be as recognized as a doctor who is, because this usually gives a doctor high exposure to other doctors. Second, there are many younger physicians that although might be a highly gifted surgeon in many procedures, have simply not been in practice long enough to have established their reputation amongst their peers. Another thing to keep in mind is that doctors who have pioneered a new procedure or technique will receive high recognition, even though there might be several unknown doctors who have become even more skillful and gifted in that procedure with time.

Because of all of these issues, we recommend you see several doctors before making the important decision. In the next chapter we will go through some of the steps you can take to help you make a well-informed decision on the plastic surgeon you choose.

We hope with the information listed in this book, it will make the important process of choosing the right plastic surgeon easier then if you didn't have this tool to start with. And ultimately that you will be very happy and satisfied with the choice you made.

Steps in choosing the right Plastic Surgeon

Although the information in this book has given you a head start in your search for a well trained and qualified surgeon, this information should never take the place of you doing your own research to make a well informed decision on a doctor. This book is only meant as a tool in that process. Below is a list of steps you can take to help guide you through the decision making process to find the right doctor.

Gathering Doctors Names

There are several ways to gather names of good plastic surgeons. Your goal should be to find a doctor who is good in the procedure you are planning to have done, just because a doctor is good at breast implants doesn't necessarily mean he or she is good at face lifts. Start by asking friends that may have had the procedure you are planning to have, ask about their experience with that doctor and how satisfied they are with the results. Another way is to ask your family doctor. He or she should be able to refer you to a good plastic surgeon, keep in mind that things change quickly in plastic surgery and your family doctor might not always have the latest up to date information to which doctor would specialize in the procedure you are looking for.

Check Credentials

ABPS - When checking board certification, it is very important to consider a doctor who is certified by the American Board of Plastic Surgery (ABPS). This assures you that this surgeon has graduated from an accredited medical school and completed at least 5 years of additional residency -

usually three years of general surgery and two years of plastic surgery. Doctors must also practice plastic surgery for two years and pass comprehensive written and oral exams to be certified by the ABPS.

Meeting the Doctor

There are several questions you will want to ask your doctors as well as things you will want to look for. We have listed some important ones below.

☑ *Check board certification and credentials!*

☑ *Ask them how many times have they performed the procedure you are planning to have done.*

☑ *Is it a specialty of theirs?*

☑ *Ask about the risks in the procedure you are seeking. Will you be put under general or local anesthesia?*

☑ *Ask to see before/after pictures of a similar situation that you will be having done. Please keep in mind doctors will usually show you their prize surgeries, request that they show you more of the same procedures then they have in their photo book.*

☑ *Ask to receive a few phone numbers to previous patients who have received the same procedure done. Take advantage of this opportunity be able to find out about the doctor's personality or bedside manner when speaking to this patient. Also ask how satisfied they are with the results and how they were treated from the office staff. The compatibility between the doctor and patient is very important not only before the surgery but more so after the surgery. It is not uncommon to have minor complications or dissatisfaction with the results. The reason for this is because you are dealing not just with the doctor's skill but with the body that likes to heal in its own way, not always the way the doctor or patient would like it to. For this reason there may need to be a second surgery to receive the desired results. There* **must** *be a comfortable and trusting relationship between doctor and patient to walk through these issues if they arise.*

☑ *Ask the doctor what you will be charged if there needs to be more surgery to receive the desired results, will you have to pay surgical center fees? Anesthesiologist fees? Nurse fees? A doctor should do these procedures for as little as possible for the patient.*

☑ *Where is the surgery done? Does the doctor have his or her in house surgical facility? If so ask if the doctor has privileges to a local hospital. To receive hospital privileges, the surgeon must first be evaluated by a hospital credentialing committee, which consists of a group of his peers.*

☑ *When asking about the fees for your surgery, if the doctor does not have an in house surgery facility, there will be a fee for the surgical center that he performs the surgery at, make sure you know what this fee will be. If the doctor will be performing it in house there may still be a fee but it will be substantially lower. If you are having a procedure that requires general anesthesia there may be an anesthesiologist fee. The doctor should be able to explain all fees to you.*

☑ *When speaking with a doctor about what changes or enhancements you are wanting done, make sure the doctor is listening to what you desire as the outcome. It is crucial that you choose a doctor who is really listening to your desires in the outcome, not a doctor who nods yes but hasn't really listened. This may be accomplished by both agreeing on the realistic desired outcome.*

Final Comments...

Although no choice you make is guaranteed, the success of your surgery begins and ends with the plastic surgeon you have chosen. So do your homework, take your time and see several surgeons, you're worth it!

NOTES

How to use this book

Voted The Best

Under each city there will be a list of procedures. Under each of those procedures there will be a list of doctors. The doctors listed first, printed in bold, and with a ϒ next to it are doctors that were chosen by their peers as being the best at that procedure.

Specialty

Listed directly under The Best will be a list of doctors who specialize in that procedure. With each survey sent out, we invited the doctors to submit a list of five procedures they knew to be their specialty, we then listed them under that specialty.

Specialty-Only Cities

The cities that are Specialy-Only listings are: Atlanta, Scottsdale, Phoenix, Seattle, Philadelphia, Boston and Las Vegas.

Because we feel we couldn't do a quality survey for these cities. We choose to do a specialty listing only. We sent out a list of twenty five procedures to ABPS Certified Plastic Surgeons throughout these cities and they were invited to choose the five procedures they knew to be their specialty. We then listed them under that procedure.

Doctor Listing by City and Specialty

Dallas
Cosmetic/Aesthetic Procedures

Breast Enlargement

♈ Fritz E. Barton, Jr. MD
Dallas Plastic Surgery Inst.
411 N. Washington, Ste. 6000
Dallas, TX 95246
Phone: (214) 821-9355

♈ Rod J. Rohrich, MD
Dept. Of Plastic Surgery
UT Southwestern Medical Ctr.
5323 Harry Hines Blvd.
Dallas, TX 75235
Phone: (214) 648-3119

♈ Vasdev S. Rai, MD
Cosmetic Surgical Ctr.
7777 Forest Lane, Ste. C-612
Dallas, TX 76280
Phone: (972) 392-3511

Robert S. Hamas, MD
8345 Walnut Hill, Ste. 120
Dallas, TX 75231
Phone: (214) 363-1073

Natan Yaker, MD
Cosmetic Surgery Assoc. Texas
4100 W. 15th St., Ste. 106
Plano, TX 75093
Phone: (972) 985-7474

Jeffrey M. Kenkel, MD
Department Of Plastic Surgery
UT Southwestern Medical Ctr.
5323 Harry Hines Blvd.
Dallas, TX 75235
Phone: (214) 648-3227

Melvyn Lerman, MD
7777 Forest Ln. Ste. B-145
Dallas, TX 75230
Phone: (972) 566-7800

H. S. Byrd, MD
Dallas Plastic Surgery Inst.
411 N. Washington Ave.
Ste. 6000 LB 13
Dallas, TX 75246
Phone: (214) 821-9662

P. Craig Hobar, MD
Dallas Plastic Surgery Inst.
411 N. Washington, Ste. 6000
Dallas, TX 75246
Phone: (214) 823-8423

Breast Lift/Breast Reduction

♈ Fritz E. Barton, Jr. MD
Dallas Plastic Surgery Inst.
411 N. Washington, Ste. 6000
Dallas, TX 95246
Phone: (214) 821-9355

♈ Jeffrey M. Kenkel, MD
Department Of Plastic Surgery
UT Southwestern Medical Ctr.
5323 Harry Hines Blvd.
Dallas, TX 75235
Phone: (214) 648-3227

♈ = Voted Best - All others are the Doctors Specialty

Dallas, cont...

Hamlet T. Newsom, MD
8220 Walnut Hill Ln. Ste. 206
Dallas, TX 75231
Phone: (214) 739-5760

Buttock Lift

♟ Rod J. Rohrich, MD
Department Of Plastic Surgery
UT Southwestern Medical Ctr.
5323 Harry Hines Blvd.
Dallas, TX 75235
Phone: (214) 648-3119

♟ C. Russell Sparenberg, MD
3900 W. 15ᵗʰ St., Ste. 106
Plano, TX 75075
Phone: (972) 867-2522

Liposuction

♟ Rod J. Rohrich, MD
Department Of Plastic Surgery
UT Southwestern Medical Ctr.
5323 Harry Hines Blvd.
Dallas, TX 75235
Phone: (214) 648-3119

♟ Jeffrey M. Kenkel, MD
Department Of Plastic Surgery
UT Southwestern Medical Ctr.
5323 Harry Hines Blvd.
Dallas, TX 75235
Phone: (214) 648-3227

Melvyn Lerman, MD
7777 Forest Ln. Ste. B-145
Dallas, TX 75230
Phone: (972) 566-7800

H. S. Byrd, MD
Dallas Plastic Surgery Inst.
411 N. Washington Ave.
Ste. 6000 LB 13
Dallas, TX 75246
Phone: (214) 821-9662

Robert S. Hamas, MD
8345 Walnut Hill, Ste. 120
Dallas, TX 75231
Phone: (214) 363-1073

Vasdev S. Rai, MD
Cosmetic Surgical Ctr.
7777 Forest Lane, Ste. C-612
Dallas, TX 76280
Phone: (972) 392-3511

P. Craig Hobar, MD
Dallas Plastic Surgery Inst.
411 N. Washington, Ste. 6000
Dallas, TX 75246
Phone: (214) 823-8423

Natan Yaker, MD
Cosmetic Surgery Assoc. Of Texas
4100 W. 15ᵗʰ St., Ste. 106
Plano, TX 75093
Phone: (972) 985-7474

Fritz E. Barton, Jr. MD
Dallas Plastic Surgery Inst.
411 N. Washington, Ste. 6000
Dallas, TX 95246
Phone: (214) 821-9355

Hamlet T. Newsom, MD
8220 Walnut Hill Ln. Ste. 206
Dallas, TX 75231
Phone: (214) 739-5760

♟ = Voted Best - All others are the Doctors Specialty

Tummy Tuck

🍸 Rod J. Rohrich, MD
Department Of Plastic Surgery
UT Southwestern Medical Ctr.
5323 Harry Hines Blvd.
Dallas, TX 75235
Phone: (214) 648-3119

Jeffrey M. Kenkel, MD
Department Of Plastic Surgery
UT Southwestern Medical Ctr.
5323 Harry Hines Blvd.
Dallas, TX 75235
Phone: (214) 648-3227

Natan Yaker, MD
Cosmetic Surgery Assoc. Of Texas
4100 W. 15th St., Ste. 106
Plano, TX 75093
Phone: (972) 985-7474

Vasdev S. Rai, MD
Cosmetic Surgical Ctr.
7777 Forest Lane, Ste. C-612
Dallas, TX 76280
Phone: (972) 392-3511

Upper Arm/Thigh Lift

🍸 Rod J. Rohrich, MD
Department Of Plastic Surgery
UT Southwestern Medical Ctr.
5323 Harry Hines Blvd.
Dallas, TX 75235
Phone: (214) 648-3119

Cheek/Chin Implants

🍸 P. Craig Hobar, MD
Dallas Plastic Surgery Inst.
411 N. Washington, Ste. 6000
Dallas, TX 75246
Phone: (214) 823-8423

Nose Surgery

🍸 Jack P. Gunter, MD
8315 Walnut Hill Lane, Ste. 225
Dallas, TX 75231
Phone: (214) 369-8123

🍸 H. S. Byrd, MD
Dallas Plastic Surgery Inst.
411 N. Washington Ave.
Ste. 6000 LB 13
Dallas, TX 75246
Phone: (214) 821-9662

🍸 Rod J. Rohrich, MD
Department Of Plastic Surgery
UT Southwestern Medical Ctr.
5323 Harry Hines Blvd.
Dallas, TX 75235
Phone: (214) 648-3119

Fritz E. Barton, Jr. MD
Dallas Plastic Surgery Inst.
411 N. Washington, Ste. 6000
Dallas, TX 95246
Phone: (214) 821-9355

Natan Yaker, MD
Cosmetic Surgery Assoc. Of Texas
4100 W. 15th St., Ste. 106
Plano, TX 75093
Phone: (972) 985-7474

🍸 = Voted Best - All others are the Doctors Specialty

Dallas, cont...

Vasdev S. Rai, MD
Cosmetic Surgical Ctr.
7777 Forest Lane
Ste. C-612
Dallas, TX 76280
Phone: (972) 392-3511

Rod J. Rohrich, MD
Department Of Plastic Surgery
UT Southwestern Medical Ctr.
5323 Harry Hines Blvd.
Dallas, TX 75235
Phone: (214) 648-3119

P. Craig Hobar, MD
Dallas Plastic Surgery Inst.
411 N. Washington, Ste. 6000
Dallas, TX 75246
Phone: (214) 823-8423

Robert S. Hamas, MD
8345 Walnut Hill, Ste. 120
Dallas, TX 75231
Phone: (214) 363-1073

Vasdev S. Rai, MD
Cosmetic Surgical Ctr.
7777 Forest Lane, Ste. C-612
Dallas, TX 76280
Phone: (972) 392-3511

Corrective Nose Surgery

♔ Jack P. Gunter, MD
8315 Walnut Hill Lane, Ste. 225
Dallas, TX 75231
Phone: (214) 369-8123

P. Craig Hobar, MD
Dallas Plastic Surgery Inst..
411 N. Washington, Ste. 6000
Dallas, TX 75246
Phone: (214) 823-8423

♔ **Rod J. Rohrich, MD**
Department Of Plastic Surgery
UT Southwestern Medical Ctr.
5323 Harry Hines Blvd.
Dallas, TX 75235
Phone: (214) 648-3119

Natan Yaker, MD
Cosmetic Surgery Assoc. Of Texas
4100 W. 15th St., Ste. 106
Plano, TX 75093
Phone: (972) 985-7474

Face Lift

Hamlet T. Newsom, MD
8220 Walnut Hill Ln.. Ste. 206
Dallas, TX 75231
Phone: (214) 739-5760

♔ **Fritz E. Barton, Jr. MD**
Dallas Plastic Surgery Inst.
411 N. Washington, Ste. 6000
Dallas, TX 95246
Phone: (214) 821-9355

H. S. Byrd, MD
Dallas Plastic Surgery Inst.
411 N. Washington Ave.
Ste. 6000 LB 13
Dallas, TX 75246
Phone: (214) 821-9662

Melvyn Lerman, MD
7777 Forest Ln. Ste. B-145
Dallas, TX 75230
Phone: (972) 566-7800

Forehead Lift

♈ Rod J. Rohrich, MD
Department Of Plastic Surgery
UT Southwestern Medical Ctr.
5323 Harry Hines Blvd.
Dallas, TX 75235
Phone: (214) 648-3119

♈ H. S. Byrd, MD
Dallas Plastic Surgery Inst.
411 N. Washington Ave.
Ste. 6000 LB 13
Dallas, TX 75246
Phone: (214) 821-9662

♈ Fritz E. Barton, Jr. MD
Dallas Plastic Surgery Inst.
411 N. Washington, Ste. 6000
Dallas, TX 95246
Phone: (214) 821-9355

♈ P. Craig Hobar, MD
Dallas Plastic Surgery Inst.
411 N. Washington, Ste. 6000
Dallas, TX 75246
Phone: (214) 823-8423

Melvyn Lerman, MD
7777 Forest Ln. Ste. B-145
Dallas, TX 75230
Phone: (972) 566-7800

Robert S. Hamas, MD
8345 Walnut Hill, Ste. 120
Dallas, TX 75231
Phone: (214) 363-1073

Eyelid Surgery

♈ H. S. Byrd, MD
Dallas Plastic Surgery Inst.
411 N. Washington Ave.
Ste. 6000 LB 13
Dallas, TX 75246
Phone: (214) 821-9662

♈ Rod J. Rohrich, MD
Department Of Plastic Surgery
UT Southwestern Medical Ctr.
5323 Harry Hines Blvd.
Dallas, TX 75235
Phone: (214) 648-3119

Fritz E. Barton, Jr. MD
Dallas Plastic Surgery Inst.
411 N. Washington, Ste. 6000
Dallas, TX 95246
Phone: (214) 821-9355

Hamlet T. Newsom, MD
8220 Walnut Hill Ln. Ste. 206
Dallas, TX 75231
Phone: (214) 739-5760

Melvyn Lerman, MD
7777 Forest Ln.. Ste. B-145
Dallas, TX 75230
Phone: (972) 566-7800

Robert S. Hamas, MD
8345 Walnut Hill, Ste. 120
Dallas, TX 75231
Phone: (214) 363-1073

Lip Enhancement

☘ Rod J. Rohrich, MD
Department Of Plastic Surgery
UT Southwestern Medical Ctr.
5323 Harry Hines Blvd.
Dallas, TX 75235
Phone: (214) 648-3119

Laser Technique

☘ A. Jay Burns, MD
5323 Harry Hines Blvd. Ste. 204
Dallas, TX 75235
Phone: (214) 648-8495

Endoscopic Technique

☘ H. S. Byrd, MD
Dallas Plastic Surgery Inst.
411 N. Washington Ave.
 Ste. 6000 LB 13
Dallas, TX 75246
Phone: (214) 821-9662

☘ Rod J. Rohrich, MD
Department Of Plastic Surgery
UT Southwestern Medical Ctr.
5323 Harry Hines Blvd.
Dallas, TX 75235
Phone: (214) 648-3119

Hand Surgery

☘ William P. Adams, MD
5323 Harry Hines Blvd.
Dallas, TX 75235
Phone: (214) 523-6835

☘ = Voted Best - All others are the Doctors Specialty

Dallas
Reconstructive Procedures

Breast Implant Removal

Y Rod J. Rohrich, MD
Department Of Plastic Surgery
UT Southwestern Medical Ctr.
5323 Harry Hines Blvd.
Dallas, TX 75235
Phone: (214) 648-3119

Y Melvyn Lerman, MD
7777 Forest Ln. Ste. B-145
Dallas, TX 75230
Phone: (972) 566-7800

Breast Reconstruction

Y Jeffrey M. Kenkel, MD
Department Of Plastic Surgery
UT Southwestern Medical Ctr.
5323 Harry Hines Blvd.
Dallas, TX 75235
Phone: (214) 648-3227

Y Hamlet T. Newsom, MD
8220 Walnut Hill Lane. Ste. 206
Dallas, TX 75231
Phone: (214) 739-5760

Y William P. Adams, MD
5323 Harry Hines Blvd
Dallas, TX 75235
Phone: (214) 523-6835

TRAM Flap Breast Reconstruction

Y Jeffrey M. Kenkel, MD
Department Of Plastic Surgery
UT Southwestern Medical Ctr.
5323 Harry Hines Blvd.
Dallas, TX 75235
Phone: (214) 648-3227

Y Hamlet T. Newsom, MD
8220 Walnut Hill Ln. Ste. 206
Dallas, TX 75231
Phone: (214) 739-5760

Y William P. Adams, MD
5323 Harry Hines Blvd
Dallas, TX 75235
Phone: (214) 523-6835

Free-Flap Breast Reconstruction

Y Jeffrey M. Kenkel, MD
Department Of Plastic Surgery
UT Southwestern Medical Ctr.
5323 Harry Hines Blvd.
Dallas, TX 75235
Phone: (214) 648-3227

Y Hamlet T. Newsom, MD
8220 Walnut Hill Ln. Ste. 206
Dallas, TX 75231
Phone: (214) 739-5760

Y William P. Adams, MD
5323 Harry Hines Blvd
Dallas, TX 75235
Phone: (214) 523-6835

Y = Voted Best - All others are the Doctors Specialty

Congenital Defects Of the Hand

♟ William P. Adams, MD
5323 Harry Hines Blvd
Dallas, TX 75235
Phone: (214) 523-6835

Cleft-Lip and Palate

♟ H.S. Byrd, MD
Dallas Plastic Surgery Institute
411 N. Washington Ave.
Ste. 6000LB 13
Dallas, TX 75246
Phone: (214) 821-9662

♟ P. Craig Hobar, MD
Dallas Plastic Surgery Inst.
411 N. Washington, Ste. 6000
Dallas, TX 75246
Phone: (214) 823-8423

Jeffrey A. Fearon, MD
The Craniofacial Ctr.
7777 Forest Lane
Dallas, TX 75230
Phone: (972) 566-6464

Ear Pinning

♟ William P. Adams, MD
5323 Harry Hines Blvd
Dallas, TX 75235
Phone: (214) 523-6835

♟ H. S. Byrd, MD
Dallas Plastic Surgery Inst.
411 N. Washington Ave.
Ste. 6000 LB 13
Dallas, TX 75246
Phone: (214) 821-9662

Jeffrey A. Fearon, MD
The Craniofacial Ctr.
7777 Forest Lane
Dallas, TX 75230
Phone: (972) 566-6464

Corrective Facial Surgery

♟ P. Craig Hobar, MD
Dallas Plastic Surgery Inst.
411 N. Washington, Ste. 6000
Dallas, TX 75246
Phone: (214) 823-8423

Jeffrey A. Fearon, MD
The Craniofacial Ctr.
7777 Forest Lane
Dallas, TX 75230
Phone: (972) 566-6464

Skin Cancer Reconstruction

♟ Rod J. Rohrich, MD
Department Of Plastic Surgery
UT Southwestern Medical Ctr.
5323 Harry Hines Blvd.
Dallas, Tx 75235
Phone: (214) 648-3119

🏆 Jeffrey M. Kenkel, MD
Department Of Plastic Surgery
UT Southwestern Medical Ctr.
5323 Harry Hines Blvd.
Dallas, TX 75235
Phone: (214) 648-3227

General Reconstruction

🏆 William P. Adams, MD
5323 Harry Hines Blvd
Dallas, TX 75235
Phone: (214) 523-6835

Craniofacial

Jeffrey A. Fearon, MD
The Craniofacial Ctr.
7777 Forest Lane
Dallas, TX 75230
Phone: (972) 566-6464

🏆 = Voted Best - All others are the Doctors Specialty

Houston
Cosmetic/Aesthetic Procedures

Breast Enlargement

℣ Jeffrey D. Friedman, MD
6560 Fannin St., Ste. 800
Houston, TX 77030
Phone: (713) 798-8188

Louis E. Walker, MD
8945 Long Point, Ste. 216
Houston, TX 77055
Phone: (713) 461-0622

Bernard Barrett, Jr. MD
Texas Inst. Of Plastic Surgery
6624 Fannin St., Ste. 2200
Houston, TX 77030
Phone: (713) 790-9000

Lisa D. Santos, MD
6624 Fannin St., Ste. 1420
Houston, TX 77030
Phone: (713) 795-0042

James F. Rosel, MD
3433 W. Alabama, Ste. D
Houston, TX 77027
Phone: (713) 961-3433

D. Robert Wiemer, MD
Wiemer Plastic Surgery
6560 Fannin St., Ste. 1760
Houston, TX 77030
Phone: (713) 795-5584

Breast Lift/Breast Reduction

Mark D. Gilliland, MD
6624 Fannin St., Ste. 2260
Houston, TX 77030
Phone: (713) 799-8885

Parviz Arfai, MD, FACS
7777 Southwest FRWY. Ste. 724
Houston, TX 77074
Phone: (713) 776-9086

D. Robert Wiemer, MD
Wiemer Plastic Surgery
6560 Fannin St., Ste. 1760
Houston, TX 77030
Phone: (713) 795-5584

David T. J. Netscher, MD
Baylor Plastic Surgery
6560 Fannin St.
Houston, TX 77030
Phone: (713) 798-5017

Bernard Barrett, Jr. MD
Texas Inst. Of Plastic Surgery
6624 Fannin St., Ste. 2200
Houston, TX 77030
Phone: (713) 790-9000

Buttock Lift

℣ Mark D. Gilliland, MD
6624 Fannin St., Ste. 2260
Houston, TX 77030
Phone: (713) 799-8885
Buttock Implants

℣ = Voted Best - All others are the Doctors Specialty

Buttock Implants

☤ Saleh M. Shenaq, MD
6560 Fannin St., Ste. 800
Houston, TX 77030
Phone: (713) 798-6310

Liposuction

☤ Mark D. Gilliland, MD
6624 Fannin St., Ste. 2260
Houston, TX 77030
Phone: (713) 799-8885

☤ Melvin Spira, MD, DDS
6560 Fannin St., Ste. 800
Houston, TX 77030
Phone: (713) 798-5227

David J. Katrana, MD, DDS
9034 W.heimer , Ste. 320
Houston, TX 77063
Phone: (713) 974-7269

Parviz Arfai, MD, FACS
7777 Southwest FRWY. Ste. 724
Houston, TX 77074
Phone: (713) 776-9086

James F. Roesel, MD
3433 W. Alabama, Ste. D
Houston, TX 77027
Phone: (713) 961-3433

Lisa D. Santos, MD
6624 Fannin St., Ste. 1420
Houston, TX 77030
Phone: (713) 795-0042

Saleh M. Shenaq, MD
6560 Fannin St., Ste. 800
Houston, TX 77030
Phone: (713) 798-6310

D. Robert Wiemer, MD
Wiemer Plastic Surgery
6560 Fannin St., Ste. 1760
Houston, TX 77030
Phone: (713) 795-5584

Mark Schusterman, MD
7505 S. Main, Ste. 200
Houston, TX 77030
Phone: (713) 794-0368

Tummy Tuck

☤ Melvin Spira, MD, DDS
6560 Fannin St., Ste. 800
Houston, TX 77030
Phone: (713) 798-5227

David J. Katrana, MD, DDS
9034 W.heimer , Ste. 320
Houston, TX 77063
Phone: (713) 974-7269

Lisa D. Santos, MD
6624 Fannin St., Ste. 1420
Houston, TX 77030
Phone: (713) 795-0042

D. Robert Wiemer, MD
Wiemer Plastic Surgery
6560 Fannin St., Ste. 1760
Houston, TX 77030
Phone: (713) 795-5584

David T. J. Netscher, MD
Baylor Plastic Surgery
6560 Fannin St.
Houston, TX 77030
Phone: (713) 798-5017

☤ = Voted Best - All others are the Doctors Specialty

Mark D. Gilliland, MD
6624 Fannin St., Ste. 2260
Houston, TX 77030
Phone: (713) 799-8885

Upper Arm/Thigh Lift

♈ Mark D. Gilliland, MD
6624 Fannin St., Ste. 2260
Houston, TX 77030
Phone: (713) 799-8885

Gifted Artistically

♈ Melvin Spira, MD, DDS
6560 Fannin St., Ste. 800
Houston, TX 77030
Phone: (713) 798-5227

♈ Steven M. Hamilton, MD
6624 Fannin St., Ste. 1650
Houston, TX 77030
Phone: (713) 797-1007

Nose Surgery

♈ Russell Kridel, MD
Facial Plastic Surgery Assoc.
1200 BINZ St., Ste. 1350
Houston, TX 77004
Phone: (713) 526-5665

♈ Samuel Stal, MD
1102 Bates, Ste. 330
Houston, TX 77030
Phone: (713) 770-3180

♈ Bernard Barrett, Jr. MD
Texas Inst. Of Plastic Surgery
6624 Fannin St., Ste. 2200
Houston, TX 77030
Phone: (713) 790-9000

Parviz Arfai, MD, FACS
7777 Southwest FRWY. Ste. 724
Houston, TX 77074
Phone: (713) 776-9086

Corrective Nose Surgery

♈ Russell Kridel, MD
Facial Plastic Surgery Assoc.
1200 BINZ St., Ste. 1350
Houston, TX 77004
Phone: (713) 526-5665

♈ Samuel Stal, MD
1102 Bates, Ste. 330
Houston, TX 77030
Phone: (713) 770-3180

Face Lift

♈ Bernard Barrett, Jr. MD
Texas Inst. Of Plastic Surgery
6624 Fannin St., Ste. 2200
Houston, TX 77030
Phone: (713) 790-9000

♈ Melvin Spira, MD, DDS
6560 Fannin St., Ste. 800
Houston, TX 77030
Phone: (713) 798-5227

David J. Katrana, MD, DDS
9034 W.heimer, Ste. 320
Houston, TX 77063
Phone: (713) 974-7269

♈ = Voted Best - All others are the Doctors Specialty

Mark D. Gilliland, MD
6624 Fannin St., Ste. 2260
Houston, TX 77030
Phone: (713) 799-8885

James F. Roesel, MD
3433 W. Alabama, Ste. D
Houston, TX 77027
Phone: (713) 961-3433

Mark Schusterman, MD
7505 S. Main, Ste. 200
Houston, TX 77030
Phone: (713) 794-0368

Lisa D. Santos, MD
6624 Fannin St., Ste. 1420
Houston, TX 77030
Phone: (713) 795-0042

D. Robert Wiemer, MD
Wiemer Plastic Surgery
6560 Fannin St., Ste. 1760
Houston, TX 77030
Phone: (713) 795-5584

Parviz Arfai, MD, FACS
7777 Southwest FRWY. Ste. 724
Houston, TX 77074
Phone: (713) 776-9086

Forehead Lift

Y Bernard Barrett, Jr. MD
Texas Inst. Of Plastic Surgery
6624 Fannin St., Ste. 2200
Houston, TX 77030
Phone: (713) 790-9000

Mark Schusterman, MD
7505 S. Main, Ste. 200
Houston, TX 77030
Phone: (713) 794-0368

Eyelid Surgery

Y Bernard Barrett, Jr. MD
Texas Inst. Of Plastic Surgery
6624 Fannin St., Ste. 2200
Houston, TX 77030
Phone: (713) 790-9000

Y James Patrinely, MD
6500 Fannin St., Ste. 1100
Houston, TX 77030
Phone: (713) 795-0705

Mark Schusterman, MD
7505 S. Main, Ste. 200
Houston, TX 77030
Phone: (713) 794-0368

Lisa D. Santos, MD
6624 Fannin St., Ste. 1420
Houston, TX 77030
Phone: (713) 795-0042

David J. Katrana, MD.
9034 W.heimer, Ste. 320
Houston, TX 77063
Phone: (713) 974-7269

James F. Roesel, MD
3433 W. Alabama, Ste. D
Houston, TX 77027
Phone: (713) 961-3433

Laser Technique

Louis E. Walker, MD
8945 Long Point, Ste. 216
Houston, TX 77055
Phone: (713) 461-0622

Y = Voted Best - All others are the Doctors Specialty

Endoscopic Technique

♈ Melvin Spira, MD, DDS
6560 Fannin St., Ste. 800
Houston, TX 77030
Phone: (713) 798-5227

Ear Pinning

♈ Samuel Stal, MD
1102 Bates, Ste. 330
Houston, TX 77030
Phone: (713) 770-3180

Spider Vein Treatment

♈ Esta Kronberg, MD
7500 Beechnut St., Ste. 228
Houston, TX 77074
Phone: (713) 771-8941

Hand Surgery

♈ David T. J. Netscher, MD
Baylor Plastic Surgery
6560 Fannin St.
Houston, TX 77030
Phone: (713) 798-5017

David W. Chang, MD
UT.MD. Anderson Cancer Ctr.
Dept. Of Plastic Surgery
Houston, TX 77030
Phone: (713) 794-1247

Louis E. Walker, MD
8945 Long Point, Ste. 216
Houston, TX 77055
Phone: (713) 461-0622

Saleh M. Shenaq, MD
6560 Fannin St., Ste. 800
Houston, TX 77030
Phone: (713) 798-6310

Houston

Reconstructive Procedures

Breast Implant Removal

℞ Franklin A. Rose, MD
Texas Inst. Of Plastic Surgery
6624 Fannin St., Ste. 2200
Houston, TX 77030
Phone: (713) 790-9000

℞ Mark Schusterman, MD
7505 S. Main, Ste. 200
Houston, TX 77030
Phone: (713) 794-0368

℞ Jeffrey D. Friedman, MD
6560 Fannin St., Ste. 800
Houston, TX 77030
Phone: (713) 798-8188

James F. Roesel, MD
3433 W. Alabama, Ste. D
Houston, TX 77027
Phone: (713) 961-3433

Breast Reconstruction

℞ Jeffrey D. Friedman, MD
6560 Fannin St., Ste. 800
Houston, TX 77030
Phone: (713) 798-8188

℞ Mark Schusterman, MD
7505 S. Main, Ste. 200
Houston, TX 77030
Phone: (713) 794-0368

℞ Stephen S. Kroll, MD
Anderson Cancer Ctr.
1515 Holcombe Blvd.
Houston, TX 77030
Phone: (713) 794-1247

Saleh M. Shenaq, MD
6560 Fannin St., Ste. 800
Houston, TX 77030
Phone: (713) 798-6310

TRAM Flap Breast Reconstruction

℞ Mark Schusterman, MD
7505 S. Main, Ste. 200
Houston, TX 77030
Phone: (713) 794-0368

℞ Stephen S. Kroll, MD
Anderson Cancer Ctr.
1515 Holcombe Blvd.
Houston, TX 77030
Phone: (713) 794-1247

℞ Jeffrey D. Friedman, MD
6560 Fannin St., Ste. 800
Houston, TX 77030
Phone: (713) 798-8188

℞ Saleh M. Shenaq, MD
6560 Fannin St., Ste. 800
Houston, TX 77030
Phone: (713) 798-6310

℞ = Voted Best - All others are the Doctors Specialty

Houston, cont...

Free-Flap Breast Reconstruction

Y Mark Schusterman, MD
7505 S. Main, Ste. 200
Houston, TX 77030
Phone: (713) 794-0368

Y Jeffrey D. Friedman, MD
6560 Fannin St., Ste. 800
Houston, TX 77030
Phone: (713) 798-8188

Y Stephen S. Kroll, MD
Anderson Cancer Ctr.
1515 Holcombe Blvd.
Houston, TX 77030
Phone: (713) 794-1247

Congenital Defects Of the Hand

Y David T. J. Netscher, MD
Baylor Plastic Surgery
6560 Fannin St.
Houston, TX 77030
Phone: (713) 798-5017

Y Fred Kessler, MD
6624 Fannin St., Ste. 2730
Houston, TX 77030
Phone: (713) 795-4950

Skin Cancer Reconstruction

Y Jeffrey D. Friedman, MD
6560 Fannin St., Ste. 800
Houston, TX 77030
Phone: (713) 798-8188

Y Stephen S. Kroll, MD
Anderson Cancer Ctr.
1515 Holcombe Blvd.
Houston, TX 77030
Phone: (713) 794-1247

David J. Katrana, MD, DDS
9034 W.heimer , Ste. 320
Houston, TX 77063
Phone: (713) 974-7269

Cleft-Lip and Palate

Y Samuel Stal, MD
1102 Bates, Ste. 330
Houston, TX 77030
Phone: (713) 770-3180

Corrective Facial Surgery

Y Samuel Stal, MD
1102 Bates, Ste. 330
Houston, TX 77030
Phone: (713) 770-3180

Saleh M. Shenaq, MD
6560 Fannin St., Ste. 800
Houston, TX 77030
Phone: (713) 798-6310

General Reconstruction

Y David T. J. Netscher, MD
Baylor Plastic Surgery
6560 Fannin St.
Houston, TX 77030
Phone: (713) 798-5017

Y = Voted Best - All others are the Doctors Specialty

David W. Chang, MD
UT.MD. Anderson Cancer Ctr.
Dept. Of Plastic Surgery
Houston, TX 77030
Phone: (713) 794-1247

Pediatric Surgery

Samuel Stal, MD
1102 Bates, Ste. 330
Houston, TX 77030
Phone: (713) 770-3180

Micro Surgery

David W. Chang, MD
UT.MD. Anderson Cancer Ctr.
Dept. Of Plastic Surgery
Houston, TX 77030
Phone: (713) 794-1247

Los Angeles Area

Cosmetic/Aesthetic Procedures

Richard Ellenbogen, MD
9201 Sunset Blvd, Ste. 202
Los Angeles, CA 90069
Phone: (310) 276-3183

Breast Lift/Breast Reduction

♈ Gareth D. Wooton, MD
1301 20th St., Ste. 470
Santa Monica, CA 90404
Phone: (310) 315-0222

Breast Enlargement

♈ D. Clavin, MD, FACS
2001 Santa Monica Blvd.
Ste. 890W
Santa Monica, CA 90404
Phone: (310) 829-5977

Armen Vartany, MD
2080 Century Park E., Ste. 604
Los Angeles, CA 90067
Phone: (310) 277-1877

Jon A. Perlman, MD
414 N. Camden Dr.
Beverly Hills, CA 90210
Phone: (310) 854-0031

Thomas S. Taylor, MD
960 East Green St., Ste. 214
Pasadena, CA 91106
Phone: (626) 577-7730

T. Gregory Kirianoff, MD
2080 Century Park East, Ste. 607
Los Angeles, CA 90067
Phone: (310) 277-4457

Anthony B. Sokol, MD
120 S. Spalding Dr., Ste. 205
Beverly Hills, CA 90212
Phone: (310) 274-8157

♈ Harvey A. Zarem, MD
1301 20th St., Ste. 470
Santa Monica, CA 90404
Phone: (310) 315-0222

Janet Salomonson, MD
2021 Santa Monica Blvd. Ste. 421E
Santa Monica, CA 90404
Phone: (310) 453-8709

Anthony B. Sokol, MD
120 S. Spalding Dr., Ste. 205
Beverly Hills, CA 90212
Phone: (310) 274-8157

Thomas S. Taylor, MD
960 East Green St., Ste. 214
Pasadena, CA 91106
Phone: (626) 577-7730

Buttock Lift

♈ Adrian Aiache, MD
9884 Little Santa Monica Blvd.
Ste. 102
Beverly Hills, CA 900212
Phone: (310) 276-5856

♈ = Voted Best - All others are the Doctors Specialty

Los Angeles, cont...

♈ Brian Novack, MD
9001 Wilshire Boulevard,
Ste. 202
Beverly Hills, CA 90211
Phone: (310) 829-9876

T. Gregory Kirianoff, MD
A Medical Corporation
2080 Century Park East, Ste. 607
Los Angeles, CA 90067
Phone: (310) 277-4457

♈ Dennis P. Thompson, MD
2001 Santa Monica Blvd.
Ste. 1180-W
Santa Monica, CA 90404
Phone: (310) 829-6876

Janet Salomonson, MD
2021 Santa Monica Blvd. Ste. 421E
Santa Monica, CA 90404
Phone: (310) 453-8709

Richard Ellenbogen, MD
9201 Sunset Blvd. Ste. 202
Los Angeles, CA 90069
Phone: (310) 276-3183

Buttock Implants

♈ Brian Novack, MD
9001 Wilshire Boulevard,
Ste. 202
Beverly Hills, CA 90211
Phone: (310) 888-8818

Anthony B. Sokol, MD
120 S. Spalding Dr., Ste. 205
Beverly Hills, CA 90212
Phone: (310) 274-8157

Liposuction

Tummy Tuck

♈ Peter Bella Fodor, MD
2080 Century Park East, Ste. 710
Los Angeles, CA 90067
Phone: (310) 203-9818

♈ Anthony B. Sokol, MD
120 S. Spalding Dr.,
Ste. 205
Beverly Hills, CA 90212
Phone: (310) 274-8157

♈ D. Clavin, MD, FACS
2001 Santa Monica Blvd.
Ste. 890W
Santa Monica, CA 90404
Phone: (310) 829-5977

Upper Arm/Thigh Lift

Cadvan Griffiths Jr. MD
11600 Wilshire Blvd. Ste. 422
Los Angeles, CA 90025
Phone: (310) 477-5558

Thomas S. Taylor, MD
960 East Green St., Ste. 214
Pasadena, CA 91106
Phone: (626) 577-7730

Jon A. Perlman, MD
414 N. Camden Dr.
Beverly Hills, CA 90210
Phone: (310) 854-0031

♈ = Voted Best - All others are the Doctors Specialty

Gifted Artistically

🏆 **D. Clavin, MD, FACS**
2001 Santa Monica Blvd.
Ste. 890W
Santa Monica, CA 90404
Phone: (310) 829-5977

Cheek/Chin Implants

🏆 **William J. Binder, MD, FACS**
9201 Sunset Blvd. Ste. 809
Los Angeles, CA 90069
Phone: (310) 858-6749

Nose Surgery

🏆 **D. Clavin, MD, FACS**
2001 Santa Monica Blvd.
Ste. 890W
Santa Monica, CA 90404
Phone: (310) 829-5977

🏆 **Richard Ellenbogen, MD**
9201 Sunset Blvd. Ste. 202
Los Angeles, CA 90069
Phone: (310) 276-3183

Armen Vartany, MD
2080 Century Park East, Ste. 604
Los Angeles, CA 90067
Phone: (310) 277-1877

T. Gregory Kirianoff, MD
A Medical Corporation
2080 Century Park East, Ste. 607
Los Angeles, CA 90067
Phone: (310) 277-4457

Corrective Nose Surgery

🏆 **D. Clavin, MD, FACS**
2001 Santa Monica Blvd.
Ste. 890W
Santa Monica, CA 90404
Phone: (310) 829-5977

🏆 **Richard Ellenbogen, MD**
9201 Sunset Blvd. Ste. 202
Los Angeles, CA 90069
Phone: (310) 276-3183

T. Gregory Kirianoff, MD
A Medical Corporation
2080 Century Park East, Ste607
Los Angeles, CA 90067
Phone: (310) 277-4457

Armen Vartany, MD
2080 Century Park East, Ste. 604
Los Angeles, CA 90067
Phone: (310) 277-1877

Face Lift

🏆 **D. Clavin, MD, FACS**
2001 Santa Monica Blvd.
Ste. 890W
Santa Monica, CA 90404
Phone: (310) 829-5977

🏆 **Gareth D. Wooton, MD**
1301 20th St., Ste. 470
Santa Monica, CA 90404
Phone: (310) 315-0222

Janet Salomonson, MD
2021 Santa Monica Blvd. Ste. 421E
Santa Monica, CA 90404
Phone: (310) 453-8709

🏆 = Voted Best - All others are the Doctors Specialty

Richard Ellenbogen, MD
9201 Sunset Blvd. Ste. 202
Los Angeles, CA 90069
Phone: (310) 276-3183

Anthony B. Sokol, MD
120 S. Spalding Dr., Ste. 205
Beverly Hills, CA 90212
Phone: (310) 274-8157

Jon A. Perlman, MD
414 N. Camden Dr.
Beverly Hills, CA 90210
Phone: (310) 854-0031

T. Gregory Kirianoff, MD
A Medical Corporation
2080 Century Park East, Ste. 607
Los Angeles, CA 90067
Phone: (310) 277-4457

Forehead Lift

♈ D. Clavin, MD, FACS
2001 Santa Monica Blvd.
Ste. 890W
Santa Monica, CA 90404
Phone: (310) 829-5977

Richard Ellenbogen, MD
9201 Sunset Blvd. Ste. 202
Los Angeles, CA 90069
Phone: (310) 276-3183

Eyelid Surgery

♈ D. Clavin, MD, FACS
2001 Santa Monica Blvd.
Ste. 890W
Santa Monica, CA 90404
Phone: (310) 829-5977

Thomas S. Taylor, MD
960 East Green St., Ste. 214
Pasadena, CA 91106
Phone: (626) 577-7730

Janet Salomonson, MD
2021 Santa Monica Blvd. Ste. 421E
Santa Monica, CA 90404
Phone: (310) 453-8709

Lip Enhancement

♈ D. Clavin, MD, FACS
2001 Santa Monica Blvd.
Ste. 890W
Santa Monica, CA 90404
Phone: (310) 829-5977

Collagen Injections

Herb Goldberg, MD
16633 Ventura Blvd. Ste. 110
Encino, CA 91436
Phone: (818) 981-3333

Scar Revision

Cadvan Griffiths Jr. MD
11600 Wilshire Blvd. Ste. 422
Los Angeles, CA 90025
Phone: (310) 477-5558

Laser Technique

♈ Robert M. Applebaum, MD
436 N. Bedford Dr., Ste. 203
Beverly Hills, CA 90210
Phone: (310) 550-7747

♈ = Voted Best - All others are the Doctors Specialty

♈ Harold A. Lancer, MD
9735 Wilshire Blvd.
Beverly Hills, CA 90212
Phone: (310) 278-8444

Thomas S. Taylor, MD
960 East Green St., Ste. 214
Pasadena, CA 91106
Phone: (626) 577-7730

Karl Stein, MD, FACS
4910 Van Nuys Blvd. Ste. 302
Sherman Oaks, CA 91403
Phone: (818) 788-9037

Endoscopic Technique

♈ Nicanor G. Isse, MD
101 S. 1st St., Ste. 200
Burbank, CA 91502
Phone: (818) 557-6595

♈ George H. Sanders, MD
16633 Ventura Blvd. Ste. 110
Encino, CA 91536
Phone: (818) 981-3333

Hand Surgery

Cadvan Griffiths, Jr. MD
11600 Wilshire Blvd. Ste. 422
Los Angeles, CA 90025
Phone: (310) 477-5558

Armen Vartany, MD
2080 Century Park East, Ste. 604
Los Angeles, CA 90067
Phone: (310) 277-1877

Neil Ford Jones, MD
200 UCLA Medical Place, Ste. 140
Los Angeles, CA 90095
Phone: (310) 794-7784

Herb Goldberg, MD
16633 Ventura Blvd. Ste. 110
Encino, CA 91436
Phone: (818) 981-3333

Ear Pinning

♈ Ruth M. Carr, MD
1301 20th St., Ste. 470
Santa Monica, CA 90404
Phone: (310) 315-0222

♈ Jeffery I. Resnick, MD
1301 20th St., Ste. 470
Santa Monica, CA 90404
Phone: (310) 315-0222

Karl Stein, MD, FACS
4910 Van Nuys Blvd. Ste. 302
Sherman Oaks, CA 91403
Phone: (818) 788-9037

♈ = Voted Best - All others are the Doctors Specialty

Los Angeles Area

Reconstructive Procedures

Breast Implant Removal

♈ D. Clavin, MD, FACS
2001 Santa Monica Blvd.
Ste. 890W
Santa Monica, CA 90404
Phone: (310) 829-5977

Herb Goldberg, MD
16633 Ventura Blvd. Ste. 110
Encino, CA 91436
Phone: (818) 981-3333

Breast Reconstruction

♈ Robert Amonic, MD
2001 Santa Monica Blvd.
Ste. 790-W
Santa Monica, CA 90404
Phone: (310) 829-7821

Herb Goldberg, MD
16633 Ventura Blvd. Ste. 110
Encino, CA 91436
Phone: (818) 981-3333

Karl Stein, MD, FACS
4910 Van Nuys Blvd. Ste. 302
Sherman Oaks, CA 91403
Phone: (818) 788-9037

TRAM Flap Breast Reconstruction

♈ William W. Shaw, MD
200 UCLA Medical Place,
Ste. 465
Los Angeles, CA 90095
Phone: (310) 825-5582

♈ Jay S. Orringer, MD
9675 Brighton Way
Beverly Hills, CA 90210
Phone: (310) 273-1663

Free-Flap Breast Reconstruction

♈ William W. Shaw, MD
200 UCLA Medical Place,
Ste. 465
Los Angeles, CA 90095
Phone: (310) 825-5582

♈ Robert Amonic, MD
2001 Santa Monica Blvd.
Santa Monica, CA 90404
Phone: (310) 829-7821

Congenital Defects of the Hand

♈ Neil Ford Jones, MD
200 UCLA Medical Place,
Ste. 140
Los Angeles, CA 90095
Phone: (310) 794-7784

Herb Goldberg, MD
16633 Ventura Blvd. Ste. 110
Encino, CA 91436
Phone: (818) 981-3333

♈ = Voted Best - All others are the Doctors Specialty

Cleft-Lip and Palate

♈ Janet Salomonson, MD
2021 Santa Monica Blvd.
Ste. 421E
Santa Monica, CA 90404
Phone: (310) 453-8709

♈ Jeffery I. Resnick, MD
1301 20ᵗʰ St., Ste. 470
Santa Monica, CA 90404
Phone: (310) 315-0222

Herb Goldberg, MD
16633 Ventura Blvd. Ste. 110
Encino, CA 91436
Phone: (818) 981-3333

General Reconstruction

Karl Stein, MD, FACS
4910 Van Nuys Blvd. Ste. 302
Sherman Oaks, CA 91403
Phone: (818) 788-9037

Corrective Facial Surgery

♈ Henry Kawamoto, Jr. MD, DDS
1301 20ᵗʰ St., Ste. 460
Santa Monica, CA 90404
Phone: (310) 829-0391

Cadvan Griffiths, Jr. MD
11600 Wilshire Blvd. Ste. 422
Los Angeles, CA 90025
Phone: (310) 477-5558

Karl Stein, MD, FACS
4910 Van Nuys Blvd. Ste. 302
Sherman Oaks, CA 91403
Phone: (818) 788-9037

Skin Cancer Reconstruction

Cadvan Griffiths, Jr. MD
11600 Wilshire Blvd. Ste. 422
Los Angeles, CA 90025
Phone: (310) 477-5558

♈ = Voted Best - All others are the Doctors Specialty

San Diego
Cosmetic/Aesthetic Procedures

Gary L. Nobel, MD
3023 Bunker Hill St., Ste. 103-A
San Diego, CA 92109
Phone: (619)272-5633

Breast Lift/Breast Reduction

☖ H. Michael Roark, MD
6386 Alvarado Court. Ste. 301
San Diego, CA 92120
Phone: (619) 229-9212

Michael J. Halls, MD
6386 Alvarado Court, Ste. 330
San Diego, CA 92120
Phone: (619) 286-6446

Breast Enlargement

☖ H. Michael Roark, MD
6386 Alvarado Court, Ste. 301
San Diego, CA 92120
Phone: (619) 229-9212

☖ James C. Pietraszek, MD
8929 University Ctr. Lane, Ste. 102
San Diego, CA 92122
Phone: (619) 450-3377

John Alexander, Sr. MD
9339 Genesee Ave. Plaza 39
San Diego, CA 92121
Phone: (619) 293-3939

Susan Kaweski, MD
Craniofacial, Reconstructive &
Cosmetic Inst.
3444 Kearny Villa Road, Ste. 401
San Diego, CA 92123
Phone: (619) 974-9876

Michael J. Halls, MD
6386 Alvarado Court, Ste. 330
San Diego, CA 92120
Phone: (619) 286-6446

Robert Singer, MD
9834 Genesse Ave. Ste. 100
La Jolla, CA 92037
Phone: (619) 455-0290

Liposuction

☖ H. Michael Roark, MD
6386 Alvarado Court, Ste. 301
San Diego, CA 92120
Phone: (619) 229-9212

☖ Ronald J. Edelson, MD
9339 Genesse Ave. Ste. P-39
San Diego, CA 92121
Phone: (619) 452-9900

Stephen M. Krant, MD
La Jolla Plastic &
Reconstructive Surgery Ctr.
528 Nautilus St.
La Jolla, CA 92037
Phone: (619) 454-3161

Robert Singer, MD
9834 Genesse Ave. Ste. 100
La Jolla, CA 92037
Phone: (619) 455-0290

☖ = Voted Best - All others are the Doctors Specialty

Michael J. Halls, MD
6386 Alvarado Court, Ste. 330
San Diego, CA 92120
Phone: (619) 286-6446

John Alexander, Sr. MD
9339 Genesee Ave. Plaza 39
San Diego, CA 92121
Phone: (619) 293-3939

Susan Kaweski, MD
Craniofacial, Reconstructive &
Cosmetic Inst.
3444 Kearny Villa Road, Ste. 401
San Diego, CA 92123
Phone: (619) 974-9876

Gifted Artistically

Y Robert Singer, MD
9834 Genesse Ave. Ste. 100
La Jolla, CA 92037
Phone: (619) 455-0290

Cheek/Chin Implants

Y H. Michael Roark, MD
6386 Alvarado Court, Ste. 301
San Diego, CA 92120
Phone: (619) 229-9212

Tummy Tuck

Y Stephen M. Krant, MD
La Jolla Plastic &
Reconstructive Surgery Ctr.
528 Nautilus St.
La Jolla, CA 92037
Phone: (619) 454-3161

John Alexander, Sr. MD
9339 Genesee Ave. Plaza 39
San Diego, CA 92121
Phone: (619) 293-3939

Gary L. Nobel, MD
3023 Bunker Hill St.
Ste. 103-A
San Diego, CA 92109
Phone: (619) 272-5633

Nose Surgery

Y Robert Singer, MD
9834 Genesse Ave. Ste. 100
La Jolla, CA 92037
Phone: (619) 455-0290

Y Stephen M. Krant, MD
La Jolla Plastic &
Reconstructive Surgery Ctr.
528 Nautilus St.
La Jolla, CA 92037
Phone: (619) 454-3161

John Alexander, Sr. MD
9339 Genesee Ave. Plaza 39
San Diego, CA 92121
Phone: (619) 293-3939

John T. Alexander, II MD
Alexander Cosmetic Surgery
9339 Genesee Ave. Plaza 39
San Diego, CA 92121
Phone: (619) 455-7557

Y = Voted Best - All others are the Doctors Specialty

Susan Kaweski, MD
Craniofacial, Reconstructive &
Cosmetic Inst.
3444 Kearny Villa Road, Ste. 401
San Diego, CA 92123
Phone: (619) 974-9876

Gary L. Nobel, MD
3023 Bunker Hill St. Ste. 103-A
San Diego, CA 92109
Phone: (619) 272-5633

Corrective Nose Surgery

♈ Stephen M. Krant, MD
La Jolla Plastic &
Reconstructive Surgery Ctr.
528 Nautilus St.
La Jolla, CA 92037
Phone: (619) 454-3161

John Alexander, Sr. MD
9339 Genesee Ave. Plaza 39
San Diego, CA 92121
Phone: (619) 293-3939

Face Lift

♈ Robert Singer, MD
9834 Genesse Ave. Ste. 100
La Jolla, CA 92037
Phone: (619) 455-0290

♈ H. Michael Roark, MD
6386 Alvarado Court, Ste. 301
San Diego, CA 92120
Phone: (619) 229-9212

Matthew C. Gleason, MD
Plastic Surgery Medical Clinic
306 Walnut Ave. Ste. 36
San Diego, CA 92103
Phone: (619) 297-4167

Gary L. Nobel, MD
3023 Bunker Hill St., Ste. 103-A
San Diego, CA 92109
Phone: (619) 272-5633

Stephen M. Krant, MD
La Jolla Plastic &
Reconstructive Surgery Ctr.
528 Nautilus St.
La Jolla, CA 92037
Phone: (619) 454-3161

Susan Kaweski, MD
Craniofacial, Reconstructive &
Cosmetic Inst.
3444 Kearny Villa Road, Ste. 401
San Diego, CA 92123
Phone: (619) 974-9876

John T. Alexander, II MD
Alexander Cosmetic Surgery
9339 Genesee Ave. Plaza 39
San Diego, CA 92121
Phone: (619) 455-7557

Michael J. Halls, MD
6386 Alvarado Court, Ste. 330
San Diego, CA 92120
Phone: (619) 286-6446

Forehead Lift

♈ Stephen M. Krant, MD
La Jolla Plastic &
Reconstructive Surgery Ctr.
528 Nautilus St.
La Jolla, CA 92037
Phone: (619) 454-3161

♈ = Voted Best - All others are the Doctors Specialty

John T. Alexander II, MD
Alexander Cosmetic Surgery
9339 Genesee Ave. Plaza 39
San Diego, CA 92121
Phone: (619) 455-7557

Eyelid Surgery

Y C. Dennis Bucko, MD, FACS
9900 Genesee Ave.
La Jolla, CA 92037
Phone: (619) 453-8484

Y Robert Singer, MD
9834 Genesse Ave. Ste. 100
La Jolla, CA 92037
Phone: (619) 455-0290

John T. Alexander II, MD
Alexander Cosmetic Surgery
9339 Genesee Ave. Plaza 39
San Diego, CA 92121
Phone: (619) 455-7557

Collagen Injections

H. Michael Roark, MD
6386 Alvarado Court, Ste. 301
San Diego, CA 92120
Phone: (619) 229-9212

Scar Revision

Y Michael J. Halls, MD
6386 Alvarado Court, Ste. 330
San Diego, CA 92120
Phone: (619) 286-6446

Hand Surgery

Y Michael J. Halls, MD
6386 Alvarado Court, Ste. 330
San Diego, CA 92120
Phone: (619) 286-6446

Y Scott W. Barttelport, MD
8929 University Ctr. Lane
San Diego, CA 92122
Phone: (619) 623-9394

Y = Voted Best - All others are the Doctors Specialty

San Diego
Reconstructive Procedures

TRAM Flap Breast Reconstruction

℀ Gilbert W. Lee, MD
3434 Midway Dr.
San Diego, CA 92110
Phone: (619) 223-4263

℀ Michael J. Halls, MD
6386 Alvarado Court, Ste. 330
San Diego, CA 92120
Phone: (619) 286-6446

Free-Flap Breast Reconstruction

℀ Michael J. Halls, MD
6386 Alvarado Court, Ste. 330
San Diego, CA 92120
Phone: (619) 286-6446

℀ Gilbert W. Lee, MD
3434 Midway Dr.
San Diego, CA 92110
Phone: (619) 223-4263

Breast Reconstruction

℀ Michael J. Halls, MD
6386 Alvarado Court, Ste. 330
San Diego, CA 92120
Phone: (619) 286-6446

℀ Gilbert W. Lee, MD
3434 Midway Dr.
San Diego, CA 92110
Phone: (619) 223-4263

Stephen M. Krant, MD
La Jolla Plastic &
Reconstructive Surgery Ctr.
528 Nautilus St.
La Jolla, CA 92037
Phone: (619) 454-3161

Congenital Defects of the Hand

℀ Michael J. Halls, MD
6386 Alvarado Court, Ste. 330
San Diego, CA 92120
Phone: (619) 286-6446

Cleft-Lip and Palate

℀ John D. Smoot, MD
9850 Genessee Ave. Ste. 3000
San Diego, CA 92037
Phone: (619) 587-9850

Corrective Facial Surgery

℗ Scott W. Barttelport, MD
8929 University Ctr. Lane
San Diego, CA 92122
Phone: (619) 623-9394

Gary L. Nobel, MD
3023 Bunker Hill St., Ste. 103-A
San Diego, CA 92109
Phone: (619) 272-5633

Skin Cancer Reconstruction

Stephen M. Krant, MD
La Jolla Plastic &
Reconstructive Surgery Ctr.
528 Nautilus St.
La Jolla, CA 92037
Phone: (619) 454-3161

General Reconstruction

℗ Jonathan W. Jones, MD
4060 4ᵗʰ Ave. Ste. 650
San Diego, CA 92103
Phone: (619) 260-1076

℗ Michael J. Halls, MD
6386 Alvarado Court, Ste. 330
San Diego, CA 92120
Phone: (619) 286-6446

℗ Gilbert W. Lee, MD
3434 Midway Dr.
San Diego, CA 92110
Phone: (619) 223-4263

Stephen M. Krant, MD
La Jolla Plastic &
Reconstructive Surgery Ctr.
528 Nautilus St.
La Jolla, CA 92037
Phone: (619) 454-3161

Craniofacial

Susan Kaweski, MD
Craniofacial, Reconstructive &
Cosmetic Inst.
3444 Kearny Villa Road, Ste. 401
San Diego, CA 92123
Phone: (619) 974-9876

℗ = Voted Best - All others are the Doctors Specialty

San Francisco Bay Area
Cosmetic/Aesthetic Procedures

Craig N. Creasman, MD
2400 Samaritan Dr., Ste. 206
San Jose, CA 95124
Phone: (408) 369-9300

John McAvoy, MD
4773 Hoen Ave.
Santa Rosa, CA 95405
Phone: (707) 526-2276

Bernard S. Alpert, MD
CPMC Davies Campus, Ste. 150
San Francisco, CA 94114
Phone: (415) 626-6644

Breast Enlargement

🏆 William Jervis, MD
1844 San Miguel Dr., Ste. 109
Walnut Creek, CA 94596
Phone: (925) 937-9700

Robert G. Aycock, MD
1855 San Miguel Dr., Ste. 4
Walnut Creek, CA 94596
Phone: (925) 937-8377

Alexander Ellenberg, MD
2550 Samaritan Dr.
San Jose, CA 95124
Phone: (408) 356-1148

R. Laurence Berkowitz, MD
3803 S. Bascom Ave. Ste. 102
Campbell, CA 95008
Phone: (408) 559-7177

Samuel N. Pearl, MD
525 S. Dr., Ste. 203
Mountain View, CA 94040
Phone: (650) 964-6600

Kevin F. Ciresi, MD
5201 Norris Canyon Road, Ste. 110
San Ramon, CA 94583
Phone: (925) 275-1685

John Q. Owsley, MD
Davies Campus CPMC
45 Castro St.
San Francisco, CA 94114
Phone: (415) 861-8040

Breast Lift/Breast Reduction

🏆 Bernard S. Alpert, MD
CPMC Davies Campus, Ste. 150
San Francisco, CA 94114
Phone: (415) 626-6644

Gary D. Salomon, MD
1580 Valencia St., Ste. 704
San Francisco, CA 94110
Phone: (415) 648-9601

Alexander Ellenberg, MD
2550 Samaritan Dr.
San Jose, CA 95124
Phone: (408) 356-1148

William Y. Hoffman, MD, FAAP
UCSF Plastic Surgery
350 Parnassus Ave. Ste. 509
San Francisco, CA 94117
Phone: (415) 476-9236

🏆 = Voted Best - All others are the Doctors Specialty

Kevin F. Ciresi, MD
5201 Norris Canyon Road, Ste. 110
San Ramon, CA 94583
Phone: (925) 275-1685

Kevin F. Ciresi, MD
5201 Norris Canyon Road, Ste. 110
San Ramon, CA 94583
Phone: (925) 275-1685

R. Laurence Berkowitz, MD
3803 S. Bascom Ave. Ste. 102
Campbell, CA 95008
Phone: (408) 559-7177

Craig N. Creasman, MD
2400 Samaritan Dr., Ste. 206
San Jose, CA 95124
Phone: (408) 369-9300

Bryant A. Toth, MD
2100 Webster St., Ste. 424
San Francisco, CA 94115
Phone: (415) 923-3008

Bryant A. Toth, MD
2100 Webster St., Ste. 424
San Francisco, CA 94115
Phone: (415) 923-3008

Robert G. Aycock, MD
1855 San Miguel Dr., Ste. 4
Walnut Creek, CA 94596
Phone: (925) 937-8377

Buttock Lift

♈ **Bryant A. Toth, MD**
2100 Webster St., Ste. 424
San Francisco, CA 94115
Phone: (415) 923-3008

Samuel N. Pearl, MD
525 S. Dr., Ste. 203
Mountain View, CA 94040
Phone: (650) 964-6600

Liposuction

Tummy Tuck

♈ **George W. Commons, MD**
1515 El Camino Real, Ste. C
Palo Alto, CA 94306
Phone: (650) 328-4570

Bernard S. Alpert, MD
CPMC Davies Campus, Ste. 150
San Francisco, CA 94114
Phone: (415) 626-6644

♈ **Gene Barrie, MD (OB/GYN)**
2299 Mowry Avenue, Ste. 3A
Fremont, CA 94538
Phone: (510) 794-1411

Ear Pinning

Gary D. Salomon, MD
1580 Valencia St., Ste. 704
San Francisco, CA 94110
Phone: (415) 648-9601

♈ **William Y. Hoffman, MD, FAAP**
UCSF Plastic Surgery
350 Parnassus Ave. Ste. 509
San Francisco, CA 94117
Phone: (415) 476-9236

♈ = Voted Best - All others are the Doctors Specialty

Gifted Artistically

❦ Hale Tolleth, MD
2425 E St., Ste. 14
Concord, CA 94520
Phone: (925) 685-4533

Bryant A. Toth, MD
2100 Webster St., Ste. 424
San Francisco, CA 94115
Phone: (415) 923-3008

Samuel N. Pearl, MD
525 S. Dr., Ste. 203
Mountain View, CA 94040
Phone: (650) 964-6600

Cheek/Chin Implants

❦ John Q. Owsley, MD
Davies Campus CPMC
45 Castro St.
San Francisco, CA 94114
Phone: (415) 861-8040

Nose Surgery

❦ Ronald P. Gruber, MD
3318 Elm St.
Oakland, CA 94609
Phone: (510) 654-9222

❦ Bernard S. Alpert, MD
CPMC Davies Campus, Ste. 150
San Francisco, CA 94114
Phone: (415) 626-6644

Robert G. Aycock, MD
1855 San Miguel Dr., Ste. 4
Walnut Creek, CA 94596
Phone: (925) 937-8377

Craig N. Creasman, MD
2400 Samaritan Dr., Ste. 206
San Jose, CA 95124
Phone: (408) 369-9300

Samuel N. Pearl, MD
525 S. Dr., Ste. 203
Mountain View, CA 94040
Phone: (650) 964-6600

John Q. Owsley, MD
Davies Campus CPMC
45 Castro St.
San Francisco, CA 94114
Phone: (415) 861-8040

Corrective Nose Surgery

❦ Ronald P. Gruber, MD
3318 Elm St.
Oakland, CA 94609
Phone: (510) 654-9222

Face Lift

❦ John Q. Owsley, MD
Davies Campus CPMC
45 Castro St.
San Francisco, CA 94114
Phone: (415) 861-8040

Bryant A. Toth, MD
2100 Webster St., Ste. 424
San Francisco, CA 94115
Phone: (415) 923-3008

Craig N. Creasman, MD
2400 Samaritan Dr., Ste. 206
San Jose, CA 95124
Phone: (408) 369-9300

❦ = Voted Best - All others are the Doctors Specialty

San Francisco, cont...

Alexander Ellenberg, MD
2550 Samaritan Dr.
San Jose, CA 95124
Phone: (408) 356-1148

Kevin F. Ciresi, MD
5201 Norris Canyon Road, Ste. 110
San Ramon, CA 94583
Phone: (925) 275-1685

Bernard S. Alpert, MD
CPMC Davies Campus, Ste. 150
San Francisco, CA 94114
Phone: (415) 626-6644

Gary D. Salomon, MD
1580 Valencia St., Ste. 704
San Francisco, CA 94110
Phone: (415) 648-9601

Robert G. Aycock, MD
1855 San Miguel Dr., Ste. 4
Walnut Creek, CA 94596
Phone: (925) 937-8377

William Y. Hoffman, MD, FAAP
UCSF Plastic Surgery
350 Parnassus Ave. Ste. 509
San Francisco, CA 94117
Phone: (415) 476-9236

John McAvoy, MD
4773 Hoen Ave.
Santa Rosa, CA 95405
Phone: (707) 526-2276

Samuel N. Pearl, MD
525 S. Dr., Ste. 203
Mountain View, CA 94040
Phone: (650) 964-6600

Forehead Lift

� John Q. Owsley, MD
Davies Campus CPMC
45 Castro St.
San Francisco, CA 94114
Phone: (415) 861-8040

Bernard S. Alpert, MD
CPMC Davies Campus, Ste. 150
San Francisco, CA 94114
Phone: (415) 626-6644

Eyelid Surgery

☙ John Q. Owsley, MD
Davies Campus CPMC
45 Castro St.
San Francisco, CA 94114
Phone: (415) 861-8040

Bryant A. Toth, MD
2100 Webster St., Ste. 424
San Francisco, CA 94115
Phone: (415) 923-3008

Craig N. Creasman, MD
2400 Sameritan Dr., Ste. 206
San Jose, CA 95124
Phone: (408) 369-9300

Alexander Ellenberg, MD
2550 Samaritan Dr.
San Jose, CA 95124
Phone: (408) 356-1148

Kevin F. Ciresi, MD
5201 Norris Canyon Road, Ste. 110
San Ramon, CA 94583
Phone: (925) 275-1685

Bernard S. Alpert, MD
CPMC Davies Campus, Ste. 150
San Francisco, CA 94114
Phone: (415) 626-6644

Y Vincent R. Hentz, MD
900 Blake Wilbur Dr.
Palo Alto, CA 94304
Phone: (650) 723-5256

Gary D. Salomon, MD
1580 Valencia St., Ste. 704
San Francisco, CA 94110
Phone: (415) 648-9601

Laser Technique

Y Issa Eshima, MD
1635 Divisadero St., Ste. 520
San Francisco, CA 94115
Phone: (415) 476-3727

Gary D. Salomon, MD
1580 Valencia St., Ste. 704
San Francisco, CA 94110
Phone: (415) 648-9601

John McAvoy, MD
4773 Hoen Ave.
Santa Rosa, CA 95405
Phone: (707) 526-2276

Endoscopic Technique

R. Laurence Berkowitz, MD
3803 S. Bascom Ave. Ste. 102
Campbell, CA 95008
Phone: (408) 559-7177

Hand Surgery

Y Kyle D. Bickel, MD
2300 California St., Ste. 300
San Francisco, CA 94115
Phone: (415) 923-0992

Y Harry J. Bunke, JR. MD
101 N. El Camino Real
San Mateo, CA 94401
Phone: (650) 342-4294

Y = Voted Best - All others are the Doctors Specialty

San Francisco Bay Area

Reconstructive Procedures

Breast Implant Removal

Ⴘ Stephen J. Mathes, MD
350 Parnassus, Ste. 509
San Francisco, CA 94117
Phone: (415) 476-3061

Alexander Ellenberg, MD
2550 Sameritan Dr.
San Jose, CA 95124
Phone: (408) 356-1148

Breast Reconstruction

Ⴘ Stephen J. Mathes, MD
350 Parnassus, Ste. 509
San Francisco, CA 94117
Phone: (415) 476-3061

Alexander Ellenberg, MD
2550 Samaritan Dr.
San Jose, CA 95124
Phone: (408) 356-1148

TRAM Flap Breast Reconstruction

Ⴘ Stephen J. Mathes, MD
350 Parnassus, Ste. 509
San Francisco, CA 94117
Phone: (415) 476-3061

Free-Flap Breast Reconstruction

Ⴘ Bernard S. Alpert, MD
CPMC Davies Campus, Ste. 150
San Francisco, CA 94114
Phone: (415) 626-6644

Ⴘ Stephen J. Mathes, MD
350 Parnassus, Ste. 509
San Francisco, CA 94117
Phone: (415) 476-3061

Ⴘ Vincent D. Lepore, Jr. MD
900 Welch Road, Ste. 110
Palo Alto, CA 94304
Phone: (650) 325-1118

Ⴘ Harry J. Bunke, JR. MD
101 N. El Camino Real
San Mateo, CA 94401
Phone: (650) 342-4294

Ⴘ Seung K. Kim, MD
900 Welch Road, Ste. 110
Palo Alto, CA 94304
Phone: (650) 325-1118

Ⴘ = Voted Best - All others are the Doctors Specialty

Congenital Defects of the Hand

Y Vincent R. Hentz, MD
900 Blake Wilbur Dr.
Palo Alto, CA 94304
Phone: (650) 723-5256

Y Harry J. Bunke, JR. MD
101 N. El Camino Real
San Mateo, CA 94401
Phone: (650) 342-8989

Cleft-Lip and Palate

Y William Y. Hoffman, MD, FAAP
UCSF Plastic Surgery
350 Parnassus Ave. Ste. 509
San Francisco, CA 94117
Phone: (415) 476-9236

R. Laurence Berkowitz, MD
3803 S. Bascom Ave. Ste. 102
Campbell, CA 95008
Phone: (408) 559-7177

Skin Cancer Reconstruction

Y Stephen J. Mathes, MD
350 Parnassus, Ste. 509
San Francisco, CA 94117
Phone: (415) 476-3061

General Reconstruction

Y Stephen J. Mathes, MD
350 Parnassus, Ste. 509
San Francisco, CA 94117
Phone: (415) 476-3061

Y Berry Press, MD
2550 Samaritan Dr., Ste. A
San Jose, CA 95124
Phone: (408) 356-1148

Pediatric Plastic Surgery

Y William Y. Hoffman, MD, FAAP
UCSF Plastic Surgery
350 Parnassus Ave. Ste. 509
San Francisco, CA 94117
Phone: (415) 476-9236

Y = Voted Best - All others are the Doctors Specialty

Miami
Cosmetic/Aesthetic Procedures

Thomas J. Zaydon Jr. MD
Cosmetic Surgery Inst. Of Miami
3661 S. Miami Ave. Ste. 509
Miami, FL 33133
Phone: (305) 856-0338

Breast Enlargement

♈ Leonard A. Roudner, MD
550 Biltmore Way, Ste. 890
Coral Gables, FL 33134
Phone: (305) 444-8585

♈ Walter R. Mullin, MD
1444 N.west 14th Ave.
Miami, FL 33125
Phone: (305) 325-1441

Joel L. Roskind, MD, FACS
7400 N. Kendall Dr., Ste. 518
Miami, FL 33156
Phone: (305) 670-1003

Gilbert B. Snyder, MD
6280 Sunset Dr.
Miami, FL 33143
Phone: (305) 666-0855

Michael E. Kelly, MD
Plastic Surgery Assoc. Of Miami
8940 N. Kendall Dr., Ste. 903E
Miami, FL 33176
Phone: (305) 595-2969

Michael D. Storch, MD
21110 Biscayne Blvd.
N. Miami Beach, FL 33180
Phone: (305) 932-3200

Breast Lift/Breast Reduction

♈ Walter R. Mullin, MD
1444 N.west 14th Ave.
Miami, FL 33125
Phone: (305) 325-1441

Thomas J. Zaydon, Jr. MD
Cosmetic Surgery Inst. Of Miami
3661 S. Miami Ave. Ste. 509
Miami, FL 33133
Phone: (305) 856-0338

John M. Cassel, MD
8950 N. Kendall Dr., Ste. 106
Miami, FL 33176
Phone: (305) 596-1010

Buttock Implants

♈ Jorge E. Hildalgo, MD
2310 and 2320 S. Dixie Hwy
Coconut Grove, FL 33133
Phone: (305) 860-0717

Liposuction

♈ Walter R. Mullin, MD
1444 N.west 14th Ave.
Miami, FL 33125
Phone: (305) 325-1441

♈ = Voted Best - All others are the Doctors Specialty

Miami, cont...

Michael D. Storch, MD
21110 Biscayne Blvd.
N. Miami Beach, FL 33180
Phone: (305) 932-3200

Darryl J. Blinski, MD
7800 Southwest 87th Ave.
Ste. C-375
Miami, FL 33173
Phone: (305) 598-0091

John M. Cassel, MD
8950 N. Kendall Dr., Ste. 106
Miami, FL 33176
Phone: (305) 596-1010

Joel L. Roskind, MD, FACS
7400 N. Kendall Dr., Ste. 518
Miami, FL 33156
Phone: (305) 670-1003

Thomas J. Zaydon, Jr. MD
Cosmetic Surgery Inst. Of Miami
3661 S. Miami Ave. Ste. 509
Miami, FL 33133
Phone: (305) 856-0338

Michael E. Kelly, MD
Plastic Surgery Assoc. Of Miami
8940 N. Kendall Dr., Ste. 903E
Miami, FL 33176
Phone: (305) 595-2969

Tummy Tuck

♈ Walter R. Mullin, MD
1444 N.west 14th Ave.
Miami, FL 33125
Phone: (305) 325-1441

Gilbert B. Snyder, MD
6280 Sunset Dr.
Miami, FL 33143
Phone: (305) 666-0855

Seth R. Thaller, MD, DMD
UMS Medical Division
Miami, FL 33101
Phone: (305) 585-5285

Joel L. Roskind, MD, FACS
7400 N. Kendall Dr., Ste. 518
Miami, FL 33156
Phone: (305) 670-1003

Michael E. Kelly, MD
Plastic Surgery Assoc. Of Miami
8940 N. Kendall Dr., Ste. 903E
Miami, FL 33176
Phone: (305) 595-2969

Nose Surgery

♈ D. Ralph Millard, Jr. MD
1444 N.west 14th Ave.
Miami, FL 33125
Phone: (305) 325-1441

♈ S. Anthony Wolfe, MD
1444 N.west 14th Ave., 2nd Floor
Miami, FL 33125
Phone: (305) 325-1300

Darryl J. Blinski, MD
7800 Southwest 87th Ave.
Ste. C-375
Miami, FL 33173
Phone: (305) 598-0091

Michael D. Storch, MD
21110 Biscayne Blvd.
N. Miami Beach, FL 33180
Phone: (305) 932-3200

Joel L. Roskind, MD, FACS
7400 N. Kendall Dr., Ste. 518
Miami, FL 33156
Phone: (305) 670-1003

♈ = Voted Best - All others are the Doctors Specialty

Gilbert B. Snyder, MD
6280 Sunset Dr.
Miami, FL 33143
Phone: (305) 666-0855

Corrective Nose Surgery

♈ D. Ralph Millard, Jr. MD
1444 N.west 14ᵗʰ Ave.
Miami, FL 33125
Phone: (305) 325-1441

♈ S. Anthony Wolfe, MD
1444 N.west 14ᵗʰ Ave., 2ⁿᵈ Floor
Miami, FL 33125
Phone: (305) 325-1300

Seth R. Thaller, MD, DMD
UMS Medical Division
Miami, FL 33101
Phone: (305) 585-5285

Thomas J. Zaydon, Jr. MD
Cosmetic Surgery Inst. Of Miami
3661 S. Miami Ave. Ste. 509
Miami, FL 33133
Phone: (305) 856-0338

Face Lift

♈ Thomas J. Baker, MD
1501 S. Miami Ave.
Miami, FL 33129
Phone: (305) 854-2424

Gilbert B. Snyder, MD
6280 Sunset Dr.
Miami, FL 33143
Phone: (305) 666-0855

Thomas J. Zaydon, Jr. MD
Cosmetic Surgery Inst. Of Miami
3661 S. Miami Ave. Ste. 509
Miami, FL 33133
Phone: (305) 856-0338

Michael D. Storch, MD
21110 Biscayne Blvd.
N. Miami Beach, FL 33180
Phone: (305) 932-3200

Walter R. Mullin, MD
1444 N.west 14ᵗʰ Ave.
Miami, FL 33125
Phone: (305) 325-1441

D. Ralph Millard, Jr. MD
1444 N.west 14ᵗʰ Ave.
Miami, FL 33125
Phone: (305) 325-1441

John M. Cassel, MD
8950 N. Kendall Dr., Ste. 106
Miami, FL 33176
Phone: (305) 596-1010

Darryl J. Blinski, MD
7800 Southwest 87ᵗʰ Ave.
Ste. C-375
Miami, FL 33173
Phone: (305) 598-0091

Michael E. Kelly, MD
Plastic Surgery Assoc. Of Miami
8940 N. Kendall Dr., Ste. 903E
Miami, FL 33176
Phone: (305) 595-2969

Eyelid Surgery

♈ Myron Tanenbaum, MD
6280 Sunset Dr., Ste. 400
S. Miami, FL 33143
Phone: (305) 662-4100

♈ = Voted Best - All others are the Doctors Specialty

Miami, cont...

John M. Cassel, MD
8950 N. Kendall Dr., Ste. 106
Miami, FL 33176
Phone: (305) 596-1010

Michael E. Kelly, MD
Plastic Surgery Assoc. Of Miami
8940 N. Kendall Dr., Ste. 903E
Miami, FL 33176
Phone: (305) 595-2969

Joel L. Roskind, MD, FACS
7400 N. Kendall Dr., Ste. 518
Miami, FL 33156
Phone: (305) 670-1003

Ear Pinning

♈ Walter R. Mullin, MD
1444 N.west 14th Ave.
Miami, FL 33125
Phone: (305) 325-1441

Seth R. Thaller, MD, DMD
UMS Medical Division
Miami, FL 33101
Phone: (305) 585-5285

Collagen Injections

♈ Alan S. Rapperport, MD
Rapperport Plastic Surgery Assoc.
6280 Sunset Dr., Ste. 501
Miami, FL 33143
Phone: (305) 666-1352

Endoscopic Technique

♈ Michael E. Kelly, MD
Plastic Surgery Assoc. Of Miami
8940 N. Kendall Dr., Ste. 903E
Miami, FL 33176
Phone: (305) 595-2969

Hand Surgery

♈ Felix M. Freshwater, MD
1150 N.west 14th St.
Miami, FL 33136
Phone: (305) 325-0600

♈ = Voted Best - All others are the Doctors Specialty

Miami

Reconstructive Procedures

Breast Implant Removal

℗ Walter R. Mullin, MD
1444 N.west 14th Ave.
Miami, FL 33125
Phone: (305) 325-1441

℗ Gilbert B. Snyder, MD
6280 Sunset Dr.
Miami, FL 33143
Phone: (305) 666-0855

TRAM Flap Breast Reconstruction

℗ Walter R. Mullin, MD
1444 N.west 14th Ave.
Miami, FL 33125
Phone: (305) 325-1441

℗ Michael E. Kelly, MD
Plastic Surgery Assoc. Of Miami
8940 N. Kendall Dr., Ste. 903E
Miami, FL 33176
Phone: (305) 595-2969

℗ John M. Cassel, MD
8950 N. Kendall Dr., Ste. 106
Miami, FL 33176
Phone: (305) 596-1010

Free-Flap Breast Reconstruction

℗ John M. Cassel, MD
8950 N. Kendall Dr., Ste. 106
Miami, FL 33176
Phone: (305) 596-1010

℗ Deirdre M. Marshall, MD
3100 Southwest 62nd Ave.
Ste. 120
Miami, FL 33155
Phone: (305) 669-6491

Breast Reconstruction

℗ John M. Cassel, MD
8950 N. Kendall Dr., Ste. 106
Miami, FL 33176
Phone: (305) 596-1010

℗ Walter R. Mullin, MD
1444 N.west 14th Ave.
Miami, FL 33125
Phone: (305) 325-1441

Michael E. Kelly, MD
Plastic Surgery Assoc. Of Miami
8940 N. Kendall Dr., Ste. 903E
Miami, FL 33176
Phone: (305) 595-2969

Congenital Defects Of the Hand

℗ Felix M. Freshwater, MD
1150 N.west 14th St.
Miami, FL 33136
Phone: (305) 325-0600

Miami, cont...

Cleft-Lip and Palate

♈ D. Ralph Millard Jr. MD
1444 N.west 14ᵗʰ Ave.
Miami, FL 33125
Phone: (305) 325-1441

Michael E. Kelly, MD
Plastic Surgery Assoc. Of Miami
8940 N. Kendall Dr., Ste. 903E
Miami, FL 33176
Phone: (305) 595-2969

Seth R. Thaller, MD, DMD
UMS Medical Division
Miami, FL 33101
Phone: (305) 585-5285

Skin Cancer Reconstruction

Michael E. Kelly, MD
Plastic Surgery Assoc. Of Miami
8940 N. Kendall Dr., Ste. 903E
Miami, FL 33176
Phone: (305) 595-2969

Corrective Facial Surgery

♈ Seth R. Thaller, MD, DMD
UMS Medical Division
Miami, FL 33101
Phone: (305) 585-5285

♈ D. Ralph Millard, Jr. MD
1444 N.west 14ᵗʰ Ave.
Miami, FL 33125
Phone: (305) 325-1441

♈ S. Anthony Wolfe, MD
1444 N.west 14ᵗʰ Ave., 2ⁿᵈ Floor
Miami, FL 33125
Phone: (305) 325-1300

General Reconstruction

♈ Felix M. Freshwater, MD
1150 N.west 14ᵗʰ St.
Miami, FL 33136
Phone: (305) 325-0600

♈ = Voted Best - All others are the Doctors Specialty

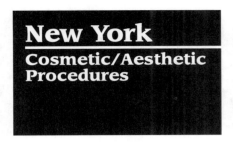

Arthur G. Ship, MD
1049 Fifth Ave. Ste. 2D
New York, NY 10028
Phone: (212) 861-8000

David L. Abramson, MD
1755 York Ave.
New York, NY 10128
Phone: (212) 426-7200

Breast Enlargement

Charles Kraft Loving, Jr. MD
17 East 84th St.
New York, NY 10028
Phone: (212) 472-0990

♈ Stephen R. Colen, MD
NYU Medical Ctr. Plastic Surgery
784 Park Ave.
New York, NY 10021
Phone: (212) 988-8900

Saul Hoffman, MD
102- East 78th St.
New York, New York 10021
Phone: (212) 734-9266

♈ Leo M. Keegan, Jr. MD
1125 Fifth Ave.
New York, NY 10028
Phone: (212) 288-9800

Robert M. Freund, MD
220 East 63rd St., Ste. LJ
New York, NY 10021
Phone: (212) 583-1200

Ronald M. Linder, MD
565 Park Ave.
New York, NY 10021
Phone: (212) 319-1717

David A. Hidalgo, MD
655 Park Ave.
New York, NY 10021
Phone: (212) 639-8991

Donald Wood Smith, MD
830 Park Ave.
New York, NY 10021
Phone: (212) 744-2224

Jane N. Haher, MD
5 East 83rd St.
New York, NY 10028
Phone: (212) 744-1828

Bryan G. Forley, MD
5 East 82nd St.
New York, NY 10028
Phone: (212) 861-3757

Stephen T. Greenberg, MD
190 Frehlich Farm Blvd.
Woodbury, NY 11297
Phone: (516) 362-7400

Carlin B. Vickery, MD
1125 Fifth Ave.
New York, NY 10021
Phone: (212) 288-9800

Steven Herman, MD
800 B 5th Avenue.
New York, NY 10021
Phone: (212) 249-7000

♈ = Voted Best - All others are the Doctors Specialty

New York City, cont...

Breast Lift/Breast Reduction

♈ Stephen R. Colen, MD
NYU Medical Ctr. Plastic Surgery
784 Park Ave.
New York, NY 10021
Phone: (212) 988-8900

♈ Saul Hoffman, MD
102- East 78th St.
New York, New York 10021
Phone: (212) 734-9266

♈ Carlin B. Vickery, MD
1125 Fifth Ave.
New York, NY 10021
Phone: (212) 288-9800

Jane N. Haher, MD
5 East 83rd St.
New York, NY 10028
Phone: (212) 744-1828

David A. Hidalgo, MD
655 Park Ave.
New York, NY 10021
Phone: (212) 639-8991

Steven Herman, MD
800 B 5th Avenue.
New York, NY 10021
Phone: (212) 249-7000

David L. Abramson, MD
1755 York Ave.
New York, NY 10128
Phone: (212) 426-7200

Liposuction

♈ Gerald H. Pitman, MD
170 East 73rd St.
New York, NY 10021
Phone: (212) 517-2600

Elliott H. Rose, MD
The Aesthetic Surgery Ctr.
895 Park Ave.
New York, NY 10021
Phone: (212) 639-1346

Lawrence S. Reed, MD
The Reed Ctr.,
45 East 85th St.
New York, NY 10021
Phone: (212) 772-8300

Bryan G. Forley, MD
5 East 82nd St.
New York, NY 10028
Phone: (212) 861-3757

Arthur G. Ship, MD
1049 Fifth Ave. Ste. 2D
New York, NY 10028
Phone: (212) 861-8000

Stephen T. Greenberg. MD
190 Frehlich Farm Blvd.
Woodbury, NY 11297
Phone: (516) 362-7400

Robert M. Freund, MD
220 East 63rd St. , Ste. LJ
New York, NY 10021
Phone: (212) 583-1200

Charles Kraft Loving, Jr. MD
17 East 84th St.
New York, NY 10028
Phone: (212) 472-0990

♈ = Voted Best - All others are the Doctors Specialty

Carlin B. Vickery, MD
1125 Fifth Ave.
New York, NY 10021
Phone: (212) 288-9800

Ronald M. Linder, MD
565 Park Ave.
New York, NY 10021
Phone: (212) 319-1717

Leo M. Keegan Jr. MD
1125 Fifth Ave.
New York, NY 10028
Phone: (212) 288-9800

Jane N. Haher, MD
5 East 83rd St.
New York, NY 10028
Phone: (212) 744-1828

Tummy Tuck

♈ Alan Matarasso, MD, FACS, PC
Plastic Surgery Facility
1009 Park Ave.
New York, NY 10028
Phone: (212) 249-7500

♈ Gerald H. Pitman, MD
170 East 73rd St.
New York, NY 10021
Phone: (212) 517-2600

Stephen T. Greenberg, MD
190 Frehlich Farm Blvd.
Woodbury, NY 11297
Phone: (516) 362-7400

Arthur G. Ship, MD
1049 Fifth Ave. Ste. 2D
New York, NY 10028
Phone: (212) 861-8000

Carlin B. Vickery, MD
1125 Fifth Ave.
New York, NY 10021
Phone: (212) 288-9800

Leo M. Keegan Jr. MD
1125 Fifth Ave.
New York, NY 10028
Phone: (212) 288-9800

Gifted Artistically

Arthur G. Ship, MD
1049 Fifth Ave. Ste. 2D
New York, NY 10028
Phone: (212) 861-8000

Cheek/Chin Implants

♈ Barry M. Zide, MD, DMD
420 East 55th St., Ste. 1-D
New York, NY 10022
Phone: (212) 421-2424

Arthur G. Ship, MD
1049 Fifth Ave. Ste. 2D
New York, NY 10028
Phone: (212) 861-8000

Nose Surgery

♈ Nicolas Tabbal, MD
521 Park Ave.
New York, NY 10021
Phone: (212) 644-5800

♈ Saul Hoffman, MD
102- East 78th St.
New York, New York 10021
Phone: (212) 734-9266

♈ = Voted Best - All others are the Doctors Specialty

Darrick E. Antell, MD
850 Park Ave.
New York, NY 10021
Phone: (212) 988-4040

Donald Wood Smith, MD
830 Park Ave.
New York, NY 10021
Phone: (212) 744-2224

Ronald M. Linder, MD
565 Park Ave.
New York, NY 10021
Phone: (212) 319-1717

Lawrence S. Reed, MD
The Reed Ctr.,
45 East 85th St.
New York, NY 10021
Phone: (212) 772-8300

Philip J. Miller, MD
530 First Ave. Ste. 3C
New York, NY 10016
Phone: (212) 263-5959

Joseph G. McCarthy, MD
722 Park Ave.
New York, NY 10021
Phone: (212) 628-4420

David A. Hidalgo, MD
655 Park Ave.
New York, NY 10021
Phone: (212) 639-8991

Bryan G. Forley, MD
5 East 82nd St.
New York, NY 10028
Phone: (212) 861-3757

Steven Herman, MD
800 B 5th Avenue.
New York, NY 10021
Phone: (212) 249-7000

Arthur G. Ship, MD
1049 Fifth Ave. Ste. 2D
New York, NY 10028
Phone: (212) 861-8000

Charles Kraft Loving Jr. MD
17 East 84th St.
New York, NY 10028
Phone: (212) 472-0990

Robert M. Freund, MD
220 East 63rd St., Ste. LJ
New York, NY 10021
Phone: (212) 583-1200

Jane N. Haher, MD
5 East 83rd St.
New York, NY 10028
Phone: (212) 744-1828

Corrective Nose Surgery

♈ Saul Hoffman, MD
102- East 78th St.
New York, New York 10021
Phone: (212) 734-9266

♈ Nicolas Tabbal, MD
521 Park Ave.
New York, NY 10021
Phone: (212) 644-5800

Robert M. Freund, MD
220 East 63rd St., Ste. LJ
New York, NY 10021
Phone: (212) 583-1200

Philip J. Miller, MD
530 First Ave. Ste. 3C
New York, NY 10016
Phone: (212) 263-5959

♈ = Voted Best - All others are the Doctors Specialty

Face Lift

Alan Matarasso, MD, FACS, PC
Plastic Surgery Facility
1009 Park Ave.
New York, NY 10028
Phone: (212) 249-7500

Sherrell J. Aston, MD
728 Park Ave.
New York, NY 10021
Phone: (212) 249-6000

David L. Abramson, MD
1755 York Ave.
New York, NY 10128
Phone: (212) 426-7200

Charles Kraft Loving, Jr. MD
17 East 84th St.
New York, NY 10028
Phone: (212) 472-0990

Joseph G. McCarthy, MD
722 Park Ave.
New York, NY 10021
Phone: (212) 628-4420

Elliott H. Rose, MD
The Aesthetic Surgery Ctr.
895 Park Ave.
New York, NY 10021
Phone: (212) 639-1346

David A. Hidalgo, MD
655 Park Ave.
New York, NY 10021
Phone: (212) 639-8991

Lawrence S. Reed, MD
The Reed Ctr.,
45 East 85th St.
New York, NY 10021
Phone: (212) 772-8300

Bryan G. Forley, MD
5 East 82nd St.
New York, NY 10028
Phone: (212) 861-3757

Arthur G. Ship, MD
1049 Fifth Ave. Ste. 2D
New York, NY 10028
Phone: (212) 861-8000

out of Business

Stephen T. Greenberg, MD
190 Frehlich Farm Blvd.
Woodbury, NY 11297
Phone: (516) 362-7400

Darrick E. Antell, MD
850 Park Ave.
New York, NY 10021
Phone: (212) 988-4040

Donald Wood Smith, MD
830 Park Ave.
New York, NY 10021
Phone: (212) 744-2224

Steven Herman, MD
800 B 5th Avenue.
New York, NY 10021
Phone: (212) 249-7000

Philip J. Miller, MD
530 First Ave. Ste. 3C
New York, NY 10016
Phone: (212) 263-5959

Leo M. Keegan, Jr. MD
1125 Fifth Ave.
New York, NY 10028
Phone: (212) 288-9800

Carlin B. Vickery, MD
1125 Fifth Ave.
New York, NY 10021
Phone: (212) 288-9800

= Voted Best - All others are the Doctors Specialty

Forehead Lift

🏆 Alan Matarasso, MD, FACS, PC
Plastic Surgery Facility
1009 Park Ave.
New York, NY 10028
Phone: (212) 249-7500

🏆 Leo M. Keegan, Jr. MD
1125 Fifth Ave.
New York, NY 10028
Phone: (212) 288-9800

Darrick E. Antell, MD
850 Park Ave.
New York, NY 10021
Phone: (212) 988-4040

Ronald M. Linder, MD
565 Park Ave.
New York, NY 10021
Phone: (212) 319-1717

Lawrence S. Reed, MD
The Reed Ctr.,
45 East 85th St.
New York, NY 10021
Phone: (212) 772-8300

Joseph G. McCarthy, MD
722 Park Ave.
New York, NY 10021
Phone: (212) 628-4420

Philip J. Miller, MD
530 First Ave. Ste. 3C
New York, NY 10016
Phone: (212) 263-5959

Eyelid Surgery

🏆 Glen W. Jelks, MD
875 Park Ave.
New York, NY 10021
Phone: (212) 988-3303

Carlin B. Vickery, MD
1125 Fifth Ave.
New York, NY 10021
Phone: (212) 288-9800

Darrick E. Antell, MD
850 Park Ave.
New York, NY 10021
Phone: (212) 988-4040

Joseph G. McCarthy, MD
722 Park Ave.
New York, NY 10021
Phone: (212) 628-4420

Philip J. Miller, MD
530 First Ave. Ste. 3C
New York, NY 10016
Phone: (212) 263-5959

Elliott H. Rose, MD
The Aesthetic Surgery Ctr.
895 Park Ave.
New York, NY 10021
Phone: (212) 639-1346

Steven Herman, MD
800 B 5th Avenue.
New York, NY 10021
Phone: (212) 249-7000

Ronald M. Linder, MD
565 Park Ave.
New York, NY 10021
Phone: (212) 319-1717

🏆 = Voted Best - All others are the Doctors Specialty

Barry M. Zide, MD, DMD
420 East 55th St., Ste. 1-D
New York, NY 10022
Phone: (212) 421-2424

Charles Kraft Loving, Jr. MD
17 East 84th St.
New York, NY 10028
Phone: (212) 472-0990

David A. Hidalgo, MD
655 Park Ave.
New York, NY 10021
Phone: (212) 639-8991

Jane N. Haher, MD
5 East 83rd St.
New York, NY 10028
Phone: (212) 744-1828

Lawrence S. Reed, MD
The Reed Ctr.,
45 East 85th St.
New York, NY 10021
Phone: (212) 772-8300

Bryan G. Forley, MD
5 East 82nd St.
New York, NY 10028
Phone: (212) 861-3757

Arthur G. Ship, MD
1049 Fifth Ave. Ste. 2D
New York, NY 10028
Phone: (212) 861-8000

Lip Enhancement

Bryan G. Forley, MD
5 East 82nd St.
New York, NY 10028
Phone: (212) 861-3757

Robert M. Freund, MD
220 East 63rd St., Ste. LJ
New York, NY 10021
Phone: (212) 583-1200

Philip J. Miller, MD
530 First Ave. Ste. 3C
New York, NY 10016
Phone: (212) 263-5959

Laser Technique

David L. Abramson, MD
1755 York Ave.
New York, NY 10128
Phone: (212) 426-7200

Stephen T. Greenberg, MD
190 Frehlich Farm Blvd.
Woodbury, NY 11297
Phone: (516) 362-7400

Endoscopic Technique

🍷 Leo M. Keegan, Jr. MD
1125 Fifth Ave.
New York, NY 10028
Phone: (212) 288-9800

Ear Pinning

🍷 Lester Silver, MD
Mt. Sinai Medical Ctr., Box 1259
1 Gustave L Levy Place
New York, NY 10029
Phone: (212) 241-5873

🍷 = Voted Best - All others are the Doctors Specialty

🏆 Court B. Cutting, MD
333 East 34th St., Ste. 1K
New York, NY 10016
Phone: (212) 263-5502

Arthur G. Ship, MD
1049 Fifth Ave. Ste. 2D
New York, NY 10028
Phone: (212) 861-8000

Hand Surgery

🏆 Robert W. Beasley, MD
310 East 30th St.
New York, NY 10016
Phone: (212) 685-3834

🏆 David T. W. Chiu, MD
161 Ft. Washington Ave. AP
Ste. 601
New York, NY 10032
Phone: (212) 305-8252

New York

Reconstructive Procedures

Saul Hoffman, MD
102- East 78th St.
New York, New York 10021
Phone: (212) 734-9266

Leo M. Keegan, Jr. MD
1125 Fifth Ave.
New York, NY 10028
Phone: (212) 288-9800

Breast Implant Removal

Y Saul Hoffman, MD
102- East 78th St.
New York, New York 10021
Phone: (212) 734-9266

Y John W. Siebert, MD
799 Park Ave.
New York, NY 10021
Phone: (212) 737-8300

Breast Reconstruction

Y Carlin B. Vickery, MD
1125 Fifth Ave.
New York, NY 10021
Phone: (212) 288-9800

Y Mark R. Sultan, MD
425 W. 59th St., Ste. 7A
New York, NY 10019
Phone: (212) 527-7277

Y David A. Hidalgo, MD
655 Park Ave.
New York, NY 10021
Phone: (212) 639-8991

TRAM Flap Breast Reconstruction

Y Mark R. Sultan, MD
425 W. 59th St., Ste. 7A
New York, NY 10019
Phone: (212) 527-7277

Y Leo M. Keegan, Jr. MD
1125 Fifth Ave.
New York, NY 10028
Phone: (212) 288-9800

Y David A. Hidalgo, MD
655 Park Ave.
New York, NY 10021
Phone: (212) 639-8991

Free-Flap Breast Reconstruction

Y Mark R. Sultan, MD
425 W. 59th St., Ste. 7A
New York, NY 10019
Phone: (212) 527-7277

Y Carlin B. Vickery, MD
1125 Fifth Ave.
New York, NY 10021
Phone: (212) 288-9800

Y = Voted Best - All others are the Doctors Specialty

New York City, cont...

♈ David A. Hidalgo, MD
655 Park Ave.
New York, NY 10021
Phone: (212) 639-8991

Congenital Defects of the Hand

♈ David T. W. Chiu, MD
161 Ft. Washington Ave.
APSte. 601
New York, NY 10032
Phone: (212) 305-8252

♈ Robert W. Beasley, MD
310 East 30ᵗʰ St.
New York, NY 10016
Phone: (212) 685-3834

Cleft-Lip and Palate

♈ Court B. Cutting, MD
333 East 34ᵗʰ St., Ste. 1K
New York, NY 10016
Phone: (212) 263-5502

♈ Lester Silver, MD
Mt. Sinai Medical Ctr., Box 1259
1 Gustave L Levy Place
New York, NY 10029
Phone: (212) 241-5873

Arthur G. Ship, MD
1049 Fifth Ave. Ste. 2D
New York, NY 10028
Phone: (212) 861-8000

Skin Cancer Reconstruction

♈ Barry M. Zide, MD, DMD
420 East 55ᵗʰ St., Ste. 1-D
New York, NY 10022
Phone: (212) 421-2424

♈ Saul Hoffman, MD
102- East 78ᵗʰ St.
New York, New York 10021
Phone: (212) 734-9266

Elliott H. Rose, MD
The Aesthetic Surgery Ctr.
895 Park Ave.
New York, NY 10021
Phone: (212) 639-1346

Corrective Facial Surgery

♈ Elliott H. Rose, MD
The Aesthetic Surgery Ctr.
895 Park Ave.
New York, NY 10021
Phone: (212) 639-1346

♈ Joseph G. McCarthy, MD
722 Park Ave.
New York, NY 10021
Phone: (212) 628-4420

General Reconstruction

♈ David T. W. Chiu, MD
161 Ft. Washington Ave.
AP Ste. 601
New York, NY 10032
Phone: (212) 305-8252

♈ = Voted Best - All others are the Doctors Specialty

Washington DC

Cosmetic/Aesthetic Procedures

Craig R. Dufrense, MD, FACS
3301 New Mexico Ave.
Washington DC 20016
Phone: (202) 966-8814

Roger Friedman, MD
5930 Hubbard Dr..
Rockville, MD 20852
Phone: (301) 881-7770

Scott L. Spear, MD
Division of Plastic Surgery
Georgetown University Medical Ctr.
3800 Reservoir Road
Washington DC 20007
Phone: (202) 687-8751

Breast Enlargement

♈ Scott L. Spear, MD
Division of Plastic Surgery
Georgetown University Medical Ctr.
3800 Reservoir Road
Washington DC 20007
Phone: (202) 687-8751

♈ Roger Friedman, MD
5930 Hubbard Dr..
Rockville, MD 20852
Phone: (301) 881-7770

Tummy Tuck

Roger Friedman, MD
5930 Hubbard Dr..
Rockville, MD 20852
Phone: (301) 881-7770

Breast Lift/Breast Reduction

♈ Scott L. Spear, MD
Division of Plastic Surgery
Georgetown University Medical Ctr.
3800 Reservoir Road
Washington DC 20007
Phone: (202) 687-8751

Gifted Artistically

♈ J. William Little, MD
1145 19th St., NW Ste. 802
Washington DC 20036
Phone: (202) 467-6700

Cheek/Chin Implants

♈ Jorge H. Reisin, MD
6410 Rockledger, Ste. 404
Bethesda, MD 20817
Phone: (301) 530-7700

Liposuction

♈ Bahman Teimourian, MD
5402 McKinley St.
Bethesda, MD 20817
Phone: (301) 897-5666

♈ = Voted Best - All others are the Doctors Specialty

Nose Surgery

Craig R. Dufrense, MD, FACS
3301 New Mexico Ave.
Washington DC 20016
Phone: (202) 966-8814

J. William Little, MD
1145 19th St., NW Ste. 802
Washington DC 20036
Phone: (202) 467-6700

Corrective Nose Surgery

♔ Craig R. Dufrense, MD, FACS
3301 New Mexico Ave.
Washington DC 20016
Phone: (202) 966-8814

J. William Little, MD
1145 19th St., NW Ste. 802
Washington DC 20036
Phone: (202) 467-6700

Face Lift

♔ J. William Little, MD
1145 19th St., NW Ste. 802
Washington DC 20036
Phone: (202) 467-6700

Roger Friedman, MD
5930 Hubbard Dr..
Rockville, MD 20852
Phone: (301) 881-7770

Craig R. Dufrense, MD, FACS
3301 New Mexico Ave.
Washington DC 20016
Phone: (202) 966-8814

Scott L. Spear, MD
Division of Plastic Surgery
Georgetown University Medical Ctr.
3800 Reservoir Road
Washington DC 20007
Phone: (202) 687-8751

Forehead Lift

♔ J. William Little, MD
1145 19th St., NW Ste. 802
Washington DC 20036
Phone: (202) 467-6700

Eyelid Surgery

Craig R. Dufrense, MD, FACS
3301 New Mexico Ave.
Washington DC 20016
Phone: (202) 966-8814

Scott L. Spear, MD
Division of Plastic Surgery
Georgetown University Medical Ctr.
3800 Reservoir Road
Washington DC 20007
Phone: (202) 687-8751

Roger Friedman, MD
5930 Hubbard Dr..
Rockville, MD 20852
Phone: (301) 881-7770

Ear Pinning

♔ Michael J. Boyajian, MD
111 Michigan Ave. NW
Washington DC, 20010
Phone: (202) 884-2157

♔ = Voted Best - All others are the Doctors Specialty

Laser Technique

Y Robert Adrian, MD
(Dermatologist)
3301 New Mexico Ave NW,
Ste. 230
Washington DC 20010
Phone: (202) 884-2157

Endoscopic Technique

Y Jorge H. Reisin, MD
6410 Rockledger, Ste404
Bethesda, MD 20817
Phone: (301) 530-7700

Spider Vein Treatment

Y Robert Adrian, MD
(Dermatologist)
3301 New Mexico Ave NW,
Ste. 230
Washington DC 20010
Phone: (202) 884-2157

Washington DC

Reconstructive Procedures

Breast Implant Removal

℣ Roger Friedman, MD
5930 Hubbard Dr..
Rockville, MD 20852
Phone: (301) 881-7770

℣ Scott L. Spear, MD
Division of Plastic Surgery
Georgetown University Medical Ctr.
3800 Reservoir Road
Washington DC 20007
Phone: (202) 687-8751

TRAM Flap Breast Reconstruction

℣ Scott L. Spear, MD
Division of Plastic Surgery
Georgetown University Medical Ctr.
3800 Reservoir Road
Washington DC 20007
Phone: (202) 687-8751

Breast Reconstruction

℣ Scott L. Spear, MD
Division of Plastic Surgery
Georgetown University Medical Ctr.
3800 Reservoir Road
Washington DC 20007
Phone: (202) 687-8751

Cleft-Lip and Palate

℣ Michael J. Boyajian, MD
111 Michigan Ave. NW
Washington DC, 20010
Phone: (202) 884-2157

℣ Jeffery Posnick, MD
5530 WI Ave. Ste. 1250
Chevy Chase, MD 20815
Phone: (301) 986-9476

Craig R. Dufrense, MD, FACS
3301 New Mexico Ave.
Washington DC 20016
Phone: (202) 966-8814

Corrective Facial Surgery

℣ Jeffery Posnick, MD
5530 WI Ave. Ste. 1250
Chevy Chase, MD 20815
Phone: (301) 986-9476

℣ Michael J. Boyajian, MD
111 Michigan Ave. NW
Washington DC, 20010
Phone: (202) 884-2157

℣ = Voted Best - All others are the Doctors Specialty

Skin Cancer Reconstruction

☥ Christopher Attinger, MD
Wound Healing Ctr.
Georgetown University Hospital
3800 Reservoir Road
Washington DC 20007
Phone: (202) 784-3307

Head and Neck Reconstruction

Christopher Attinger, MD
Wound Healing Ctr.
Georgetown University Hospital
3800 Reservoir Road
Washington DC 20007
Phone: (202) 784-3307

General Reconstruction

☥ Christopher Attinger, MD
Wound Healing Ctr.
Georgetown University Hospital
3800 Reservoir Road
Washington DC 20007
Phone: (202) 784-3307

Lower Extremity Reconstruction

Christopher Attinger, MD
Wound Healing Ctr.
Georgetown University Hospital
3800 Reservoir Road
Washington DC 20007
Phone: (202) 784-3307

Micro Surgery

Christopher Attinger, MD
Wound Healing Ctr.
Georgetown University Hospital
3800 Reservoir Road
Washington DC 20007
Phone: (202) 784-3307

Atlanta
Cosmetic/Aesthetic Procedures

Breast Enlargement

Frank Elliott, MD
Atlanta Plastic Surgery
975 Johnson Ferry Road, Ste. 500
Atlanta, GA 30347
Phone: (404) 256-1311

T. Roderick Hester, Jr. MD
Paces Plastic Surgery &
Recovery Ctr.
3200 Downwood Circle, Ste. 640
Atlanta, GA 30327
Phone: (404) 351-0051

William E. Silver, MD, FACS
4553 N. Shallowford Road, Ste. 20B
Atlanta, GA 30338
Phone: (770) 457-6303

Fredrick T. Work, MD
Atlanta Plastic Surgery
2001 Peachtree St., Ste. 545
Atlanta, GA 30306
Phone: (404) 351-1155

Robert E. Zaworski, MD
N.side Ctr. For Plastic Surgery
980 Johnson Ferry Road, Ste. 450
Atlanta, GA 30342
Phone: (404) 851-9576

Breast Lift/Breast Reduction

T. Roderick Hester, Jr. MD
Paces Plastic Surgery &
Recovery Ctr.
3200 Downwood Circle, Ste. 640
Atlanta, GA 30327
Phone: (404) 351-0051

Dianne C. Leeb, MD
3103 Fielding Dr.
Atlanta, GA 30345
Phone: (770) 491-1151

B. Alfred Phil, MD
3130 Fielding Dr.
Atlanta, GA 30345
Phone: (770) 491-1151

Frank Elliott, MD
Atlanta Plastic Surgery
975 Johnson Ferry Road, Ste. 500
Atlanta, GA 30347
Phone: (404) 256-1311

Fredrick T. Work, MD
Atlanta Plastic Surgery
2001 Peachtree St., Ste. 545
Atlanta, GA 30306
Phone: (404) 351-1155

Liposuction

T. Roderick Hester, Jr. MD
Paces Plastic Surgery &
Recovery Ctr.
3200 Downwood Circle, Ste. 640
Atlanta, GA 30327
Phone: (404) 351-0051

Atlanta, cont...

Dianne C. Leeb, MD
3103 Fielding Dr.
Atlanta, GA 30345
Phone: (770) 491-1151

B. Alfred Phil, MD
3130 Fielding Dr.
Atlanta, GA 30345
Phone: (770) 491-1151

William E. Silver, MD, FACS
4553 N. Shallowford Road, Ste. 20B
Atlanta, GA 30338
Phone: (770) 457-6303

Frank Elliott, MD
Atlanta Plastic Surgery
975 Johnson Ferry Road, Ste. 500
Atlanta, GA 30347
Phone: (404) 256-1311

Brow Lift

Dianne C. Leeb, MD
3103 Fielding Dr.
Atlanta, GA 30345
Phone: (770) 491-1151

T. Roderick Hester, Jr. MD
Paces Plastic Surgery &
Recovery Ctr.
3200 Downwood Circle, Ste. 640
Atlanta, GA 30327
Phone: (404) 351-0051

Nose Surgery

William E. Silver, MD, FACS
4553 N. Shallowford Road, Ste. 20B
Atlanta, GA 30338
Phone: (770) 457-6303

Face Lift

Dianne C. Leeb, MD
3103 Fielding Dr.
Atlanta, GA 30345
Phone: (770) 491-1151

Frank Elliott, MD
Atlanta Plastic Surgery
975 Johnson Ferry Road, Ste. 500
Atlanta, GA 30347
Phone: (404) 256-1311

Robert E. Zaworski, MD
N.side Ctr. For Plastic Surgery
980 Johnson Ferry Road, Ste. 450
Atlanta, GA 30342
Phone: (404) 851-9576

T. Roderick Hester, Jr. MD
Paces Plastic Surgery &
Recovery Ctr.
3200 Downwood Circle, Ste. 640
Atlanta, GA 30327
Phone: (404) 351-0051

Fredrick T. Work, MD
Atlanta Plastic Surgery
2001 Peachtree St., Ste. 545
Atlanta, GA 30306
Phone: (404) 351-1155

William E. Silver, MD, FACS
4553 N. Shallowford Road, Ste. 20B
Atlanta, GA 30338
Phone: (770) 457-6303

℞ = Voted Best - All others are the Doctors Specialty

B. Alfred Phil, MD
3130 Fielding Dr.
Atlanta, GA 30345
Phone: (770) 491-1151Forehead Lift

Dianne C. Leeb, MD
3103 Fielding Dr.
Atlanta, GA 30345
Phone: (770) 491-1151

Fredrick T. Work, MD
Atlanta Plastic Surgery
2001 Peachtree St., Ste. 545
Atlanta, GA 30306
Phone: (404) 351-1155

Tummy Tuck

Fredrick T. Work, MD
Atlanta Plastic Surgery
2001 Peachtree St., Ste. 545
Atlanta, GA 30306
Phone: (404) 351-1155

Eyelid Surgery

B. Alfred Phil, MD
3130 Fielding Dr.
Atlanta, GA 30345
Phone: (770) 491-1151

Dianne C. Leeb, MD
3103 Fielding Dr.
Atlanta, GA 30345
Phone: (770) 491-1151

T. Roderick Hester, Jr. MD
Paces Plastic Surgery &
Recovery Ctr.
3200 Downwood Circle, Ste. 640
Atlanta, GA 30327
Phone: (404) 351-0051

Robert E. Zaworski, MD
N.side Ctr. For Plastic Surgery
980 Johnson Ferry Road, Ste. 450
Atlanta, GA 30342
Phone: (404) 851-9576

Frank Elliott, MD
Atlanta Plastic Surgery
975 Johnson Ferry Road, Ste. 500
Atlanta, GA 30347
Phone: (404) 256-1311

Laser Technique

William E. Silver, MD, FACS
4553 N. Shallowford Road, Ste. 20B
Atlanta, GA 30338
Phone: (770) 457-6303

T. Roderick Hester, Jr. MD
Paces Plastic Surgery &
Recovery Ctr.
3200 Downwood Circle, Ste. 640
Atlanta, GA 30327
Phone: (404) 351-0051

Dianne C. Leeb, MD
3103 Fielding Dr.
Atlanta, GA 30345
Phone: (770) 491-1151

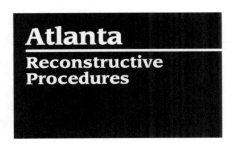

Atlanta
Reconstructive Procedures

Breast Reconstruction

Frank Elliott, MD
Atlanta Plastic Surgery
975 Johnson Ferry Road, Ste. 500
Atlanta, GA 30347
Phone: (404) 256-1311

Fredrick T. Work, MD
Atlanta Plastic Surgery
2001 Peachtree St., Ste. 545
Atlanta, GA 30306
Phone: (404) 351-1155

Corrective Facial Surgery

Robert E. Zaworski, MD
N.side Ctr. For Plastic Surgery
980 Johnson Ferry Road, Ste. 450
Atlanta, GA 30342
Phone: (404) 851-9576

Las Vegas
Cosmetic/Aesthetic Procedures

Walter G. Sullivan, MD
500 S. Rancho Dr., Ste. 8-B
Las Vegas', NV 89106
Phone: (702) 259-7759

Breast Enlargement

Stephen W. Weiland, MD
The Weiland Group
653 Town Ctr. Dr., Ste. 108
Las Vegas, NV 89134
Phone: (702) 254-0500

Walter G. Sullivan, MD
500 S. Rancho Dr., Ste. 8-B
Las Vegas', NV 89106
Phone: (702) 259-7759

William A. Zamboni, MD
Ctr. for Excellence in Plastic Surgery
1707 W. Charleston Blvd. Ste. 190
Las Vegas, NV 89102
Phone: (702) 671-5110

Liposuction

William A. Zamboni, MD
Ctr. for Excellence in Plastic Surgery
1707 W. Charleston Blvd. Ste. 190
Las Vegas, NV 89102
Phone: (702) 671-5110

Stephen W. Weiland, MD
The Weiland Group
653 Town Ctr. Dr., Ste. 108
Las Vegas, NV 89134
Phone: (702) 254-0500

Tummy Tuck

Walter G. Sullivan, MD
500 S. Rancho Dr., Ste. 8-B
Las Vegas', NV 89106
Phone: (702) 259-7759

Stephen W. Weiland, MD
The Weiland Group
653 Town Ctr. Dr., Ste. 108
Las Vegas, NV 89134
Phone: (702) 254-0500

Gifted Artistically

Joseph J. Bongiovi, MD
2121 E. Flamingo Road, Ste. 200
Las Vegas, NV 89119
Phone: (702) 733-7070

Nose Surgery

Joseph J. Bongiovi, MD
2121 E. Flamingo Road, Ste. 200
Las Vegas, NV 89119
Phone: (702) 733-7070

Face Lift

Stephen W. Weiland, MD
The Weiland Group
653 Town Ctr. Dr., Ste. 108
Las Vegas, NV 89134
Phone: (702) 254-0500

Y = Voted Best - All others are the Doctors Specialty

Walter G. Sullivan, MD
500 S. Rancho Dr., Ste. 8-B
Las Vegas', NV 89106
Phone: (702) 259-7759

Joseph J. Bongiovi, MD
2121 E. Flamingo Road, Ste. 200
Las Vegas, NV 89119
Phone: (702) 733-7070

William A. Zamboni, MD
Ctr. for Excellence in Plastic Surgery
1707 W. Charleston Blvd. Ste. 190
Las Vegas, NV 89102
Phone: (702) 671-5110

Laser Technique

William A. Zamboni, MD
Ctr. for Excellence in Plastic Surgery
1707 W. Charleston Blvd. Ste. 190
Las Vegas, NV 89102
Phone: (702) 671-5110

Endoscopic Technique

Joseph J. Bongiovi, MD
2121 E. Flamingo Road, Ste. 200
Las Vegas, NV 89119
Phone: (702) 733-7070

Forehead Lift

Joseph J. Bongiovi, MD
2121 E. Flamingo Road, Ste. 200
Las Vegas, NV 89119
Phone: (702) 733-7070

Eyelid Surgery

Stephen W. Weiland, MD
The Weiland Group
653 Town Ctr. Dr., Ste. 108
Las Vegas, NV 89134
Phone: (702) 254-0500

Brow Lift

William A. Zamboni, MD
Ctr. for Excellence in Plastic Surgery
1707 W. Charleston Blvd. Ste. 190
Las Vegas, NV 89102
Phone: (702) 671-5110

Y = Voted Best - All others are the Doctors Specialty

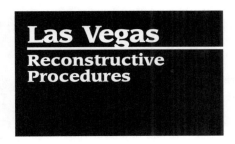

Las Vegas
Reconstructive Procedures

Cleft-Lip and Palate

Walter G. Sullivan, MD
500 S. Rancho Dr., Ste. 8-B
Las Vegas, NV 89106
Phone: (702) 259-7759

MediaPerspectives

Scottsdale Arizona

Cosmetic/Aesthetic Procedures

Breast Lift/Breast Reduction

William D. Leighton, MD
10210 N. 92nd St., Ste. 200
Scottsdale, AZ 85258
Phone: (602) 314-2008

Paul L. Schnur, MD
13400 E. Shea Blvd.
Scottsdale, AZ 85259
Phone: (602) 301-8139

Breast Enlargement

Richard D. Anderson, MD
10210 N. 92nd St.
Scottsdale, AZ 85258
Phone: (602) 860-9333

Gregory J. Mackay, MD
13400 E. Shea Blvd.
Scottsdale, AZ 85259
Phone: (602) 301-8074

Paul L. Schnur, MD
13400 E. Shea Blvd.
Scottsdale, AZ 85259
Phone: (602) 301-8139

Deborah Trojanowski, MD
3501 N. Scottsdale Road., Ste. 348
Scottsdale, AZ 85251
Phone: (602) 481-0133

John J. Corey, MD
10210 N. 92nd St., Ste. 200
Scottsdale, AZ 85258
Phone: (602) 314-2008

Deborah J. White, MD
Edwards Professional Park II
8952 E. Desert Cove, Ste. 110
Scottsdale, AZ 85260
Phone: (602) 614-3535

Deborah Trojanowski, MD
3501 N. Scottsdale Road, Ste. 348
Scottsdale, AZ 85251
Phone: (602) 481-0133

Liposuction

Deborah J. White, MD
Edwards Professional Park II
8952 E. Desert Cove, Ste. 110
Scottsdale, AZ 85260
Phone: (602) 614-3535

Gregory J. Mackay, MD
13400 E. Shea Blvd.
Scottsdale, AZ 85259
Phone: (602) 301-8074

Paul L. Schnur, MD
13400 E. Shea Blvd.
Scottsdale, AZ 85259
Phone: (602) 301-8139

Y = Voted Best - All others are the Doctors Specialty

Tummy Tuck

John J. Corey, MD
10210 N. 92nd St., Ste. 200
Scottsdale, AZ 85258
Phone: (602) 314-2008

Deborah J. White, MD
Edwards Professional Park II
8952 E. Desert Cove, Ste. 110
Scottsdale, AZ 85260
Phone: (602) 614-3535

Gifted Artistically

Deborah J. White, MD
Edwards Professional Park II
8952 E. Desert Cove, Ste. 110
Scottsdale, AZ 85260
Phone: (602) 614-3535

Richard D. Anderson, MD
10210 N. 92nd St.
Scottsdale, AZ 85258
Phone: (602) 860-9333

Cheek/Chin Implants

John J. Corey, MD
10210 N. 92nd St., Ste. 200
Scottsdale, AZ 85258
Phone: (602) 314-2008

Richard D. Anderson, MD
10210 N. 92nd St.
Scottsdale, AZ 85258
Phone: (602) 860-9333

Nose Surgery

John J. Corey, MD
10210 N. 92nd St., Ste. 200
Scottsdale, AZ 85258
Phone: (602) 314-2008

Ronald E. Barnes, MD
3300 N. 75th St.
Scottsdale, AZ 85251
Phone: (602) 990-8808

Face Lift

Gregory J. Mackay, MD
13400 E. Shea Blvd.
Scottsdale, AZ 85259
Phone: (602) 301-8074

Ronald E. Barnes, MD
3300 N. 75th St.
Scottsdale, AZ 85251
Phone: (602) 990-8808

William D. Leighton, MD
10210 N. 92nd St., Ste. 200
Scottsdale, AZ 85258
Phone: (602) 314-2008

Richard D. Anderson, MD
10210 N. 92nd St.
Scottsdale, AZ 85258
Phone: (602) 860-9333

Deborah Trojanowski, MD
3501 N. Scottsdale Road, Ste. 348
Scottsdale, AZ 85251
Phone: (602) 481-0133

Paul L. Schnur, MD
13400 E. Shea Blvd.
Scottsdale, AZ 85259
Phone: (602) 301-8139

Y = Voted Best - All others are the Doctors Specialty

Forehead Lift

Ronald E. Barnes, MD
3300 N. 75th St.
Scottsdale, AZ 85251
Phone: (602) 990-8808

William D. Leighton, MD
10210 N. 92nd St., Ste. 200
Scottsdale, AZ 85258
Phone: (602) 314-2008

Endoscopic Technique

Ronald E. Barnes, MD
3300 N. 75th St.
Scottsdale, AZ 85251
Phone: (602) 990-8808

Richard D. Anderson, MD
10210 N. 92nd St.
Scottsdale, AZ 85258
Phone: (602) 860-9333

Eyelid Surgery

John J. Corey, MD
10210 N. 92nd St., Ste. 200
Scottsdale, AZ 85258
Phone: (602) 314-2008

Richard D. Anderson, MD
10210 N. 92nd St.
Scottsdale, AZ 85258
Phone: (602) 860-9333

Hand Surgery

Deborah Trojanowski, MD
3501 N. Scottsdale Road, Ste. 348
Scottsdale, AZ 85251
Phone: (602) 481-0133

Laser Technique

Richard D. Anderson, MD
10210 N. 92nd St.
Scottsdale, AZ 85258
Phone: (602) 860-9333

Ronald E. Barnes, MD
3300 N. 75th St.
Scottsdale, AZ 85251
Phone: (602) 990-8808

Scottsdale Arizona
Reconstructive Procedures

Skin Cancer Reconstruction

Paul L. Schnur, MD
13400 E. Shea Blvd.
Scottsdale, AZ 85259
Phone: (602) 301-8139

Burn Reconstruction

William D. Leighton, MD
10210 N. 92nd St., Ste. 200
Scottsdale, AZ 85258
Phone: (602) 314-2008

Breast Reconstruction

Deborah J. White, MD
Edwards Professional Park II
8952 E. Desert Cove, Ste. 110
Scottsdale, AZ 85260
Phone: (602) 614-3535

Gregory J. Mackay, MD
13400 E. Shea Blvd.
Scottsdale, AZ 85259
Phone: (602) 301-8074

William D. Leighton, MD
10210 N. 92nd St., Ste. 200
Scottsdale, AZ 85258
Phone: (602) 314-2008

General Reconstruction

John J. Corey, MD
10210 N. 92nd St., Ste. 200
Scottsdale, AZ 85258
Phone: (602) 314-2008

Craniofacial Disorders

Gregory J. Mackay, MD
13400 E. Shea Blvd.
Scottsdale, AZ 85259
Phone: (602) 301-8074

TRAM Flap Breast Reconstruction

William D. Leighton, MD
10210 N. 92nd St., Ste. 200
Scottsdale, AZ 85258
Phone: (602) 314-2008

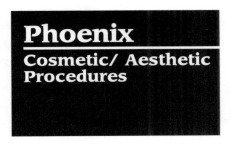

Phoenix
Cosmetic/ Aesthetic Procedures

John Ward, MD
5090 N. 40ᵗʰ St., Ste. 150
Phoenix, AZ 85018
Phone: (602) 553-0888

Jack A. Friendland, MD
101 E. Coronado Road
Phoenix, AZ 85004
Phone: (602) 257-8480

Breast Enlargement

Sood Suchart, MD
6036 N. 19ᵗʰ Ave. Ste. 311
Phoenix, AZ 85015
Phone: (602) 242-4804

Jack A. Friendland, MD
101 E. Coronado Road
Phoenix, AZ 85004
Phone: (602) 257-8480

John W. Bass, MD
16620 N. 40ᵗʰ St., Building F
Phoenix, AZ 85032
Phone: (602) 485-1010

John Ward, MD
5090 N. 40ᵗʰ St., Ste. 150
Phoenix, AZ 85018
Phone: (602) 553-0888

Liposuction

John W. Bass, MD
16620 N. 40ᵗʰ St., Building F
Phoenix, AZ 85032
Phone: (602) 485-1010

Sood Suchart, MD
6036 N. 19ᵗʰ Ave. Ste. 311
Phoenix, AZ 85015
Phone: (602) 242-4804

Tummy Tuck

Sood Suchart, MD
6036 N. 19ᵗʰ Ave. Ste. 311
Phoenix, AZ 85015
Phone: (602) 242-4804

John W. Bass, MD
16620 N. 40ᵗʰ St.
Building F
Phoenix, AZ 85032
Phone: (602) 485-1010

John Ward, MD
5090 N. 40ᵗʰ St., Ste. 150
Phoenix, AZ 85018
Phone: (602) 553-0888

Cheek/Chin Implants

Sood Suchart, MD
6036 N. 19ᵗʰ Ave. Ste. 311
Phoenix, AZ 85015
Phone: (602) 242-4804

Y = Voted Best - All others are the Doctors Specialty

Corrective Nose Surgery

Jack A. Friendland, MD
101 E. Coronado Road
Phoenix, AZ 85004
Phone: (602) 257-8480

Face Lift

Jack A. Friendland, MD
101 E. Coronado Road
Phoenix, AZ 85004
Phone: (602) 257-8480

Sood Suchart, MD
6036 N. 19th Ave. Ste. 311
Phoenix, AZ 85015
Phone: (602) 242-4804

Neck Lift

John W. Bass, MD
16620 N. 40th St., Building F
Phoenix, AZ 85032
Phone: (602) 485-1010

Forehead Lift

Sood Suchart ,MD
6036 N. 19th Ave. Ste. 311
Phoenix, AZ 85015
Phone: (602) 242-4804

John W. Bass, MD
16620 N. 40th St., Building F
Phoenix, AZ 85032
Phone: (602) 485-1010

Jack A. Friendland, MD
101 E. Coronado Road
Phoenix, AZ 85004
Phone: (602) 257-8480

Eyelid Surgery

Sood Suchart, MD
6036 N. 19th Ave. Ste. 311
Phoenix, AZ 85015
Phone: (602) 242-4804

John Ward, MD
5090 N. 40th St., Ste. 150
Phoenix, AZ 85018
Phone: (602) 553-0888

Laser Technique

Sood Suchar, MD
6036 N. 19th Ave. Ste. 311
Phoenix, AZ 85015
Phone: (602) 242-4804

John Ward, MD
5090 N. 40th St., Ste. 150
Phoenix, AZ 85018
Phone: (602) 553-0888

Endoscopic Technique

John Ward, MD
5090 N. 40th St., Ste. 150
Phoenix, AZ 85018
Phone: (602) 553-0888

℣ = Voted Best - All others are the Doctors Specialty

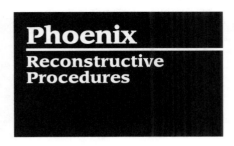

Phoenix

Reconstructive Procedures

Breast Implant Removal

Jack A. Friendland, MD
101 E. Coronado Road
Phoenix, AZ 85004
Phone: (602) 257-8480

Breast Reconstruction

Jack A. Friendland, MD
101 E. Coronado Road
Phoenix, AZ 85004
Phone: (602) 257-8480

Cleft-Lip and Palate

Jack A. Friendland, MD
101 E. Coronado Road
Phoenix, AZ 85004
Phone: (602) 257-8480

NOTES

Seattle
Cosmetic/Aesthetic Procedures

Robert M. Grenley, MD
600 Broadway, Ste. 320
Seattle, WA 98122
Phone: (206) 324-1120

Phil Haeck, MD
901 Boren Ave. Ste. 1650
Seattle, WA 98104
Phone: (206) 464-0873

Breast Enlargement

Robert M. Grenley, MD
600 Broadway, Ste. 320
Seattle, WA 98122
Phone: (206) 324-1120

Phil Haeck, MD
901 Boren Ave. Ste. 1650
Seattle, WA 98104
Phone: (206) 464-0873

Curran J. Smith, MD
1221 Madison St., Ste. 1102
Seattle, WA 98104
Phone: (206) 682-8137

Breast Lift/Breast Reduction

Robert M. Grenley, MD
600 Broadway, Ste. 320
Seattle, WA 98122
Phone: (206) 324-1120

Liposuction

Curran J. Smith, MD
1221 Madison St., Ste. 1102
Seattle, WA 98104
Phone: (206) 682-8137

Tummy Tuck

Curran J. Smith, MD
1221 Madison St., Ste. 1102
Seattle, WA 98104
Phone: (206) 682-8137

Robert M. Grenley, MD
600 Broadway, Ste. 320
Seattle, WA 98122
Phone: (206) 324-1120

Nose Surgery

Curran J. Smith, MD
1221 Madison St., Ste. 1102
Seattle, WA 98104
Phone: (206) 682-8137

Face Lift

Robert M. Grenley, MD
600 Broadway, Ste. 320
Seattle, WA 98122
Phone: (206) 324-1120

Phil Haeck, MD
901 Boren Ave. Ste. 1650
Seattle, WA 98104
Phone: (206) 464-0873

℥ = Voted Best - All others are the Doctors Specialty

Curran J. Smith, MD
1221 Madison St., Ste. 1102
Seattle, WA 98104
Phone: (206) 682-8137

Eyelid Surgery

Phil Haeck, MD
901 Boren Ave. Ste. 1650
Seattle, WA 98104
Phone: (206) 464-0873

Laser Technique

Phil Haeck, MD
901 Boren Ave. Ste. 1650
Seattle, WA 98104
Phone: (206) 464-0873

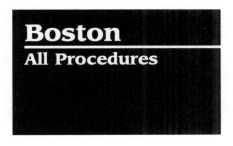

Breast Reconstruction

Fouad J. Samaha, MD, FACS
2100 Dorchester Ave. Ste. 2201
Boston, MA 02124
Phone: (617) 296-5551

Breast Enlargement

Joseph A. Russo, MD
575 Boylston St.
Newton Centre, MA 02459
Phone: (617) 964-1440

Fouad J. Samaha, MD, FACS
2100 Dorchester Ave. Ste. 2201
Boston, MA 02124
Phone: (617) 296-5551

Francis G. Wolfort, MD
110 Francis St.
Boston, MA 02275
Phone: (617) 632-8039

Breast Lift/Breast Reduction

Francis G. Wolfort, MD
110 Francis St.
Boston, MA 02275
Phone: (617) 632-8039

Fouad J. Samaha, MD, FACS
2100 Dorchester Ave. Ste. 2201
Boston, MA 02124
Phone: (617) 296-5551

Liposuction

Fouad J. Samaha, MD, FACS
2100 Dorchester Ave. Ste. 2201
Boston, MA 02124
Phone: (617) 296-5551

Joseph A. Russo, MD
575 Boylston St.
Newton Centre, MA 02459
Phone: (617) 964-1440

Tummy Tuck

Joseph A. Russo, MD
575 Boylston St.
Newton Centre, MA 02459
Phone: (617) 964-1440

Fouad J. Samaha, MD, FACS
2100 Dorchester Ave. Ste. 2201
Boston, MA 02124
Phone: (617) 296-5551

Gifted Artistically

G. Gregory Gallico III, MD
275 Cambridge St.
Boston, MA 02114
Phone: (617) 724-6900

Facelift

G. Gregory Gallico III, MD
275 Cambridge St.
Boston, MA 02114
Phone: (617) 724-6900

Francis G. Wolfort, MD
110 Francis St.
Boston, MA 02275
Phone: (617) 632-8039

Joseph A. Russo, MD
575 Boylston St.
Newton Centre, MA 02459
Phone: (617) 964-1440

Forehead Lift

G. Gregory Gallico III, MD
275 Cambridge St.
Boston, MA 02114
Phone: (617) 724-6900

Eyelid Surgery

Francis G. Wolfort, MD
110 Francis St.
Boston, MA 02275
Phone: (617) 632-8039

G. Gregory Gallico III, MD
275 Cambridge St.
Boston, MA 02114
Phone: (617) 724-6900

Cheek/Chin Implants

G. Gregory Gallico III, MD
275 Cambridge St.
Boston, MA 02114
Phone: (617) 724-6900

Nose Surgery

Joseph A. Russo, MD
575 Boylston St.
Newton Centre, MA 02459
Phone: (617) 964-1440

G. Gregory Gallico III, MD
275 Cambridge St.
Boston, MA 02114
Phone: (617) 724-6900

Francis G. Wolfort, MD
110 Francis St.
Boston, MA 02275
Phone: (617) 632-8039

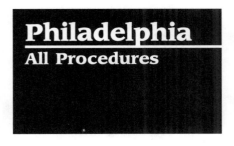

Philadelphia
All Procedures

Breast Enlargement

Charles D. Long, MD
3300 Henry Ave.
Philadelphia, PA 19129
Phone: (215) 842-7600

Richard P. Glunk, MD, FACS
100 Lancaster Ave. Ste. 660
Philadelphia, PA 19151
Phone: (610) 354-8800

Algird R. Mameniskis, MD
255South 17th St., Ste. 2200
Philadelphia, PA 19103
Phone: (215) 732-3340

Howard S. Caplan, MD
The Curtis Ctr., Ste. 506 E.
Independence Square W.
Philadelphia, PA 19106
Phone: (215) 629-1866

Francine A. Cedrone, MD
17B Industrial Blvd. Ste. 102
Paoli, PA 19301
Phone: (610) 647-2608

John H. Moore, Jr. MD
210 W. Rittenhouse Square
Philadelphia, PA 19103
Phone: (215) 546-2100

Breast Lift/Breast Reduction

Carl H. Manstein, MD
7500 Central Ave. Ste. 210
Philadelphia, PA 19111
Phone: (215) 742-6700

Algird R. Mameniskis, MD
255South 17th St., Ste. 2200
Philadelphia, PA 19103
Phone: (215) 732-3340

Francine A. Cedrone, MD
17B Industrial Blvd. Ste. 102
Paoli, PA 19301
Phone: (610) 647-2608

Howard S. Caplan, MD
The Curtis Ctr., Ste. 506 E.
Independence Square W.
Philadelphia, PA 19106
Phone: (215) 629-1866

Breast Reconstruction

Charles D. Long, MD
3300 Henry Ave.
Philadelphia, PA 19129
Phone: (215) 842-7600

Liposuction

Richard P. Glunk, MD, FACS
100 Lancaster Ave. Ste. 660
Philadelphia, PA 19151
Phone: (610) 354-8800

Philadelphia, cont...

John H. Moore, Jr. MD
210 W. Rittenhouse Square
Philadelphia, PA 19103
Phone: (215) 546-2100

Algird R. Mameniskis, MD
255South 17th St., Ste. 2200
Philadelphia, PA 19103
Phone: (215) 732-3340

Charles D. Long, MD
3300 Henry Ave.
Philadelphia, PA 19129
Phone: (215) 842-7600

Howard S. Caplan, MD
The Curtis Ctr., Ste. 506 E.
Independence Square W.
Philadelphia, PA 19106
Phone: (215) 629-1866

Francine A. Cedrone, MD
17B Industrial Blvd. Ste. 102
Paoli, PA 19301
Phone: (610) 647-2608

Algird R. Mameniskis, MD
255South 17th St., Ste. 2200
Philadelphia, PA 19103
Phone: (215) 732-3340

Tummy Tuck

John H. Moore, Jr. MD
210 W. Rittenhouse Square
Philadelphia, PA 19103
Phone: (215) 546-2100

Howard S. Caplan, MD
The Curtis Ctr., Ste. 506 E.
Independence Square W.
Philadelphia, PA 19106
Phone: (215) 629-1866

Francine A. Cedrone, MD
17B Industrial Blvd. Ste. 102
Paoli, PA 19301
Phone: (610) 647-2608

Algird R. Mameniskis, MD
255South 17th St., Ste. 2200
Philadelphia, PA 19103
Phone: (215) 732-3340

Gifted Artistically

Richard P. Glunk, MD, FACS
100 Lancaster Ave. Ste. 660
Philadelphia, PA 19151
Phone: (610) 354-8800

Face lift

Richard P. Glunk, MD, FACS
100 Lancaster Ave. Ste. 660
Philadelphia, PA 19151
Phone: (610) 354-8800

Howard S. Caplan, MD
The Curtis Ctr., Ste. 506 E.
Independence Square W.
Philadelphia, PA 19106
Phone: (215) 629-1866

Francine A. Cedrone, MD
17B Industrial Blvd. Ste. 102
Paoli, PA 19301
Phone: (610) 647-2608

♟ = Voted Best - All others are the Doctors Specialty

John H. Moore, Jr. MD
210 W. Rittenhouse Square
Philadelphia, PA 19103
Phone: (215) 546-2100

Charles D. Long, MD
3300 Henry Ave.
Philadelphia, PA 19129
Phone: (215) 842-7600

Eyelid Surgery

John H. Moore, Jr. MD
210 W. Rittenhouse Square
Philadelphia, PA 19103
Phone: (215) 546-2100

Cheek/Chin Implants

John H. Moore JR MD
210 W. Rittenhouse Square
Philadelphia, PA 19103
Phone: (215) 546-2100

Nose Surgery

Carl H. Manstein, MD
7500 Central Ave. Ste. 210
Philadelphia, PA 19111
Phone: (215) 742-6700

Algird R. Mameniskis, MD
255 S. 17th St., Ste. 2200
Philadelphia, PA 19103
Phone: (215) 732-3340

Richard P. Glunk, MD, FACS
100 Lancaster Ave. Ste. 660
Philadelphia, PA 19151
Phone: (610) 354-8800

Corrective Nose Surgery

Carl H. Manstein, MD
7500 Central Ave. Ste. 210
Philadelphia, PA 19111
Phone: (215) 742-6700

Skin Cancer Reconstruction

Charles D. Long, MD
3300 Henry Ave.
Philadelphia, PA 19129
Phone: (215) 842-7600

Carl H. Manstein, MD
7500 Central Ave. Ste. 210
Philadelphia, PA 19111
Phone: (215) 742-6700

Ear Pinning Surgery

Carl H. Manstein, MD
7500 Central Ave. Ste. 210
Philadelphia, PA 19111
Phone: (215) 742-6700

𝕐 = Voted Best - All others are the Doctors Specialty